PERSONALITY DISORDERS

PERSONALITY DISORDERS

Elements, History, Examples, and Research

VERA SONJA MAASS

Health and Psychology
Sourcebooks

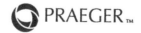 PRAEGER™

An Imprint of ABC-CLIO, LLC
Santa Barbara, California • Denver, Colorado

Library of Congress Cataloging-in-Publication Data

Names: Maass, Vera Sonja, author.
Title: Personality disorders : elements, history, examples, and research /
  Vera Sonja Maass.
Description: Santa Barbara, California : Praeger, 2019. | Series: Health and
  psychology sourcebooks | Includes bibliographical references and index.
Identifiers: LCCN 2018039665 | ISBN 9781440860454 (hardcopy : alk. paper) |
  ISBN 9781440860461 (ebook)
Subjects: LCSH: Personality disorders.
Classification: LCC RC554 .M223 2019 | DDC 616.85/81—dc23
LC record available at https://lccn.loc.gov/2018039665

ISBN: 978-1-4408-6045-4 (print)
      978-1-4408-6046-1 (ebook)

23 22 21 20 19   2 3 4 5

This book is also available as an eBook.

Praeger
An Imprint of ABC-CLIO, LLC

ABC-CLIO, LLC
147 Castilian Drive
Santa Barbara, California 93117
www.abc-clio.com

This book is printed on acid-free paper ∞

Manufactured in the United States of America

Contents

Series Foreword

An understanding of both physical diseases and mental disorders is vital to each of us, as sicknesses of body and mind touch every one of us throughout our lives—personally; among family, friends, and associates; and in our immediate and greater society. Yet the cacophony of existing information sources—from piecemeal and poorly sourced Web sites to dense academic tomes—can make acquiring accurate, accessible, and objective facts a complicated venture. This series is a solution to that dilemma.

The Health and Psychology Sourcebooks series addresses physical, psychological, and environmental conditions that threaten human health and well-being. These books are designed to accessibly and reliably fulfill the needs of students and researchers at community and undergraduate college levels, whether they are seeking vetted information for core or elective courses, papers and publications, or personal enlightenment.

Each volume presents a topic in health or psychology and explains the symptoms, diagnosis, incidence, development, causes, treatments, and related theory. "Up Close" vignettes illustrate how the disease or disorder and its associated difficulties present in various people and scenarios. History and classic as well as emerging research are detailed. Where controversy is present, it is discussed. Each volume also offers a glossary of terms, references, and resources for further reading.

Introduction

In the early 1980s, personality disorder was apparently not always considered a legitimate topic for behavioral research, judging by the fact that a speaker at a conference about cognitive behavioral approaches purposely did not explicitly mention the topic of his talk within the title for fear of being criticized (Pretzer, 1994). Yet studies that were conducted during the 1980s about the effects of personality disorder on the cognitive treatment of other mental disorders revealed discouraging results (Giles, 1985; Turner, 1987). When patients with a diagnosis of personality disorder were included, poorer outcomes were noted.

One way of looking at personality disorder is to consider its functional aspects. As stated by Gordon Allport some 80 years ago, "Personality is something and personality does something" (1937, p. 48) The implication is that personality's function is to solve major life tasks—problems individuals are confronted with in everyday life (Cantor, 1990). Thus, focusing on the functional aspects as a basis, personality disorder may be interpreted as the "failure to arrive at solutions to life tasks" (Livesley et al., 1994).

Other views see the modern concept of personality disorder as two connected notions. One notion is based on the thought that the personality abnormality causes problems for the stricken individual and/or others. The alternative thought holds that the behavior is so antisocial as to be dangerous to society. Within the classification of personality disorders, the clinical definitions range from the most timid (avoidant, dependent) to the most dangerous (antisocial) of human beings (Castillo, 2003).

No single psychosocial or biological factor causes a personality disorder; instead, the cumulative effects of multiple factors—each one only having a small effect—give rise to the disorder.

Psychological, genetic, and environmental factors each contribute to the development of personality disorders. As is commonly assumed, adverse life experiences, such as familial dysfunction, traumatic experiences, and social stresses, constitute important etiological factors as indicated by research (Paris, 2001). Genetic factors raise important implications of a different kind, such as questions about the extent to which personality can change and what kinds of change can be expected as results of treatment. Because genes are generally associated with individual traits rather than with categories of disorder, and single genes are not associated with broad personality dimensions, the biological mechanisms behind overt symptoms—what have been called "endophenotypes"—need to be examined (Gottesman & Gould, 2003). Genes interact with other genes and are turned on and off by the environment (Rutter, 2006). Their effects can only be understood by studying interactions between genetic vulnerability and life stressors (Caspi et al., 2003).

Although internal personality dynamics might seem to play the primary role in maintaining maladaptive and symptomatic behavior, reality demonstrates that much of the stability of behavior depends on consistencies in the environment. In other words, much of the stability in individuals' personalities is dependent on their environments remaining the same (Caspi & Bem, 1990). Stable social networks and enduring relationships within the frameworks of regular events, occurring frequently, tend to evoke similar responses and consistent behaviors in individuals, leading to impressions of internal stability and continuity.

The untreatability of personality disorders has been a widely held belief in the past, as demonstrated in the study "The Patients Psychiatrists Dislike" (Lewis & Appleby, 1988).

Regardless of the nature of the origins of personality disorders, they are mental health conditions that affect how individuals with these conditions think, perceive, feel about, or relate to others in their environment. The American Psychiatric Association's *Diagnostic and Statistical Manual of Mental Disorders* identifies 10 personality disorders, which are grouped into three categories or "clusters." The clusters are based on common behaviors observed in people with personality disorders.

Cluster A is characterized by odd or eccentric behaviors and includes paranoid (suspiciousness of others' motives), schizoid (detachment from social relationships and normal emotions), and schizotypal (acute discomfort in close relationships combined with distorted perceptions and eccentric behavior) personality disorders.

Cluster B is characterized by dramatic, emotional, or erratic behaviors. This category includes antisocial (disregard for society's norms and other people), borderline (pervasive instability in moods and emotions, lack of strong identity, chronic impulsive behavior), histrionic (extreme emotions and attention-seeking behaviors), and narcissistic (grandiosity, egocentric behavior, need for admiration) personality disorders.

Cluster C is characterized by anxiety and fearfulness and includes avoidant (social inhibition, hypersensitivity, feelings of inadequacy), dependent (inability and/or unwillingness to take care of oneself or make decisions), and obsessive-compulsive (preoccupation with orderliness and perfectionism) personality disorders (Bjornlund, 2011).

References

Allport, G. W. (1937). *Personality: A psychological interpretation.* New York, NY: Holt, Rinehart & Winston.

Bjornlund, L. (2011). *Personality disorders.* San Diego, CA: Reference Point Press.

Cantor, N. (1990). From thought to behavior: "Having" and "doing" in the study of personality and cognition. *American Psychologist, 45,* 735–750.

Caspi, A., & Bem, D. J. (1990). Personality continuity and change across the life course. In L. A. Pervin (Ed.), *Handbook of personality: Theory and research* (pp. 549–575). New York, NY: Guilford Press.

Caspi, A., Sugden, K., Moffitt, T. E., Taylor, A., Craig, I. W., Harrington, H., ... Poulton, R. (2003). Influence of life stress on depression: Moderation by a polymorphism in the 5-HTT gene. *Science, 301,* 386–389.

Castillo, H. (2003). *Personality disorder—temperament or trauma?* Philadelphia: Jessica Kingsley Publishers.

Giles, T. (1985). Behavioral treatment of severe bulimia. *Behavior Therapy, 16,* 393–405.

Gottesman, I. I., & Gould, T. D. (2003). The endophenotype concept in psychiatry: etymology and strategic intentions. *The American Journal of Psychiatry, 160*(4), 636–645.

Lewis, G., & Appleby, L. (1988). Personality disorder: the patients psychiatrists dislike. *The British Journal of Psychiatry, 153*(1), 44–49.

Livesley, W. J., Schroeder, M. L., Jackson, D. N., & Jang, K. L. (1994). Categorical distinctions in the study of personality disorder: Implications for classification. *Journal of Abnormal Psychology, 103*(1), 6–17.

Paris, J. (2001). Psychosocial adversity. In W. J. Livesley (Ed.), *Handbook of personality disorders: Theory, research, and treatment* (pp. 231–241). New York, NY: Guilford Press.

Pretzer, J. (1994). Cognitive therapy of personality disorders: The state of the art. *American Journal of Clinical Psychology and Psychotherapy, 1*(5), 257–266.

Rutter, M. (2006). *Genes and behavior: Nature-nurture interplay explained.* London: Blackwell.

Turner, R. (1987). The effects of personality disorder diagnosis on the outcome of social anxiety symptom reduction. *Journal of Personality Disorders, 1,* 136–143.

CHAPTER 1

Antisocial Personality Disorder

Symptoms, Diagnosis, and Incidence

Antisocial personality disorder (ASPD) presents a particularly challenging type of personality disorder, as it is characterized by impulsive, irresponsible, and often criminal behavior (NHS Choices). In the *Diagnostic and Statistical Manual of Mental Disorders* (*DSM-5*), the list of diagnostic criteria for the definition of ASPD (within Cluster B personality disorders) includes failure to conform to social norms with respect to lawful behaviors; deceitfulness, such as repeated lying, use of aliases, and conning others for personal profit or pleasure; impulsivity or failure to plan ahead; irritability and aggressiveness, as indicated by repeated physical fights; reckless disregard for safety of self or others; consistent irresponsibility, such as failure to sustain consistent work behavior or honor financial obligations; and lack of remorse, evidenced by indifference about or rationalizing mistreatment of others.

These behaviors usually start in childhood or early adolescence, often leading to a diagnosis of conduct disorder, and—being manifested in many life areas—they continue into adulthood (Goodwin & Guze, 1989). Conduct disorder prior to age 15 is a prelude to the adult condition of ASPD (Bayer, 2000).

It is noteworthy that the pattern of ASPD has also been referred to as *psychopathy*, *sociopathy*, or *dissocial personality disorder* (see the discussion of Diagnostic Features section in *DSM-5*). The term *sociopathy* may be utilized by sociologists when referring to the spectrum of low/no conscience disorders that are related to learned behavior as opposed to innate pathological tendencies that psychopaths are born with (Brown, 2009).

However, opinions differ, and some do not consider sociopathy to be a personality disorder or a formal psychiatric condition. Instead, sociopathy is thought by some to refer to patterns of attitudes and behaviors that are considered antisocial and criminal by society at large but are regarded as normal or even necessary by the subculture or social environment in which they developed. In other words, sociopaths may in fact possess a well-developed conscience and a normal capacity for empathy, guilt, and loyalty, but their loyalty and their sense of right and wrong are based on the norms and expectations of their subculture or group (Babiak & Hare, 2006).

As emphasized by experts, it is important to note that within a psychiatric context, the term *antisocial* has nothing to do with a person's ability to socialize, and it is not a description of those who are shy, inhibited, reclusive, or withdrawn. Rather, the term implies a rebellion against society, a denial of individuals' obligations to one another. This should be kept in mind while discussing this disorder (Black, 2013).

Criminal and antisocial behaviors play a major role in the definition of ASPD as listed in the American Psychiatric Association's *Diagnostic and Statistical Manual of Mental Disorders (DSM-5)*, and in this sense, ASPD is similar to sociopathy. Some individuals diagnosed with ASPD are psychopaths, but many are not. The difference between ASPD and psychopathy, as some researchers explain, is that psychopathy includes personality traits such as lack of empathy, grandiosity, and shallow emotion—traits that are not requirements for a diagnosis of ASPD (Babiak & Hare, 2006).

The *DSM-5* makes a connection between ASPD, sociopathy, dissocial personality, and psychopathy, which has given rise to some confusion within the scientific community. As the overall goal of this book is to include rather than exclude important information, available relevant data and findings pertaining to the various classifications discussed above are reported here.

The *DSM-5* reports 12-month prevalence rates of ASPD as falling between 0.2 percent and 3.3 percent, with the highest prevalence (greater than 70%) found among severe samples.

Studies with adult populations in the United States have shown prevalence rates of 3.6 to 4 percent, with males significantly outnumbering females (Compton et al., 2005; Black, 2013; Wood, 2010).

Timeline

1801   Philippe Pinel spoke of "manie sans delire" (mania without delirium).

1835   English physician James Prichard coined the term "moral insanity" to explain the difference between willful behavior that violates social norms and traditional notions of madness.

1891   German physician Julius Koch introduced the term psycho-pathic *inferiority*.

1904   The Royal Commission on the Care and Control of the Feeble Minded proposed that the "moral imbecile" should become an additional category of patients to whom care and control should be extended.

1905   Kraepelin replaced *inferiority* with *personality* and defined the psychopathic personality, which included seven types.

1913   The "Moral Defective" became a category incorporated into the Mental Deficiency Act.

1932   Schneider, a German psychiatrist, extended the classification of psychopathy to include 10 subclassifications.

1939   Scottish psychiatrist David Henderson defined three types of psychopaths: the predominantly inadequate psychopath, the predominantly aggressive psychopath, and the creative psychopath.

1941   Hervey Cleckley described psychopathic personality characteristics in his book *The Mask of Sanity: An Attempt to Reinterpret the So-Called Psychopathic Personality*, officially replaced by sociopathic personality.

1968   The designation "sociopathic personality" was replaced by "personality disorder, antisocial type." The words "sociopath" and "antisocial" refer to reactions against society and rejection of its rules and obligations (Black, 2013).

1980   The designation was changed to "antisocial personality disorder" in *DSM-III*.

1991   Robert Hare developed the Psychopathy Checklist (Revised), PCL-R.

History

In the early 19th century, French psychiatrist Philippe Pinel observed patients exhibiting explosive and irrational violence while, at the same time, seeming to understand their actions and surroundings. They did not display delusions and hallucinations generally associated with insanity. Pinel used the term "manie sans delire"—mania without delirium—to describe his observations (Black, 2013).

In 1835 English physician James Prichard formulated a new term, *moral insanity*, to define a morbid perversion of the natural human feelings (Castillo, 2003).

Physician Benjamin Rush, founder of Pennsylvania Hospital, the first psychiatric facility in the United States, and signer of the Declaration of Independence, expanded on Pinel's work by describing habitual, deliberate bad behavior and suggesting a cause that anticipated the findings of neuroscience research nearly two centuries later (Craft, 1966; Black, 2013).

Although Prichard's concept of moral insanity aided in the understanding of recurrent antisocial behavior, the term itself did not stick. Toward the end of the 19th century, a group of German psychiatrists led by Julius Koch introduced the term *psychiatric inferiority*, indicating the behavior was a reaction against society and a rejection of its rules and obligations. Later, in 1905, Kraepelin replaced *psychiatric inferiority* with *psychopathic personality* and defined within it seven types: excitable, unstable, eccentric, liars, swindlers, antisocial, and quarrelsome.

In 1932, Schneider, another German psychiatrist, extended the classification of psychopathy to include 10 subcategories, incorporating not only persons who caused suffering to others but also those who caused suffering to themselves, and not necessarily others. Schneider's theory included not just dissocial characteristics but a much wider meaning incorporating personality abnormalities of all types (Castillo, 2003).

Popularization of the word *psychopathic* occurred through the efforts of two authors working independently. In 1939 David Henderson, a Scottish psychiatrist, published the book *Psychopathic States*, in which he defined three types of psychopaths: aggressive, inadequate, and creative.

However, it was Henderson's U.S. contemporary, psychiatrist Hervey Cleckley, who developed what is considered to be the first coherent description of antisocial personality in his now classic book *The Mask of Sanity*, which was originally published in 1941 and has been revised four times since then.

Cleckley defined the condition as a disorder distinct from other psychiatric problems, viewing it as a constellation of 16 traits that define the psychopath. He added that the disorder, as he described it, should never be considered an excuse for misbehavior (Black, 2013).

Both Cleckley's and Henderson's ideas were incorporated into the first *Diagnostic and Statistical Manual of Mental Disorders (DSM-I)*, published in 1952 and representing the first formal effort by the American Psychiatric Association to catalogue in one volume the different disorders listed (Black, 2013).

With the second edition of the *DSM* in 1968, the term *antisocial personality disorder* was introduced, giving the condition an identity separate from the addictions and deviant sexuality. It took more than a decade to develop diagnostic criteria for the disorders that were introduced in *DSM-III*, published in 1980.

Development and Causes

In searching for the origin or cause of ASPD, the issue of heredity versus environment is usually raised. Some attempts to answer the question are seen in the debate surrounding the issue of whether or not sociopathy and psychopathy are the same disorders. The debate seems to reflect the users' views about the origin and determinants of the clinical syndrome. Those who believe that the condition that leads individuals to act antisocially is forged entirely by social and environmental forces call it *sociopathy*. Others, who are convinced that the condition is derived from a combination of psychological, biological, and genetic factors—or a combination of genetics, the makeup of the brain, and environment—prefer the term *psychopathy* (Hare, 1993; McGregor & McGregor, 2014; Kiehl, 2014).

Bestowing a name on a disorder does not determine its origin or cause. Various twin studies and adoption studies have been designed to find answers. In reality, adopted as well as biological children of antisocial parents face an increased risk of having this disorder, but it is thought that due to the genetic component, ASPD occurs more often among close relatives of people who have the disorder (female members are at an even greater risk than males). Biological relatives of individuals with ASPD are also more likely to develop substance-abuse disorders and somatization disorder (medical symptoms related to psychological ills; Bayer, 2000).

Several twin studies provide evidence that genetic factors play at least as important a role in the development of the disorder. A longitudinal study investigating sociopathic traits and their absence in 3,226 pairs of male twins found that eight sociopathic symptoms were heritable (Stout, 2005). Conversely, some forensic psychiatrists, when focusing on the many factors involved in the cause of ASPD, may consider maternal deprivation during the child's first five years, leading to insufficient nurturing and socialization in addition to having an antisocial or alcoholic father (even if he is not in residence), to be an important factor in the development of the disorder (Simon, 1996).

In the case of sociopaths, sociologists believe that the disorder is acquired through learned conditioning, such as exposure to pathological environments (Brown, 2009). Others see part of the cause in today's highly mobile society, wherein individual accountability to family,

community, and moral standards has been diminished, which may present fewer restraints in relatively anonymous urban settings with transient populations, making it easier to act out negative impulses without
intervention from community members (Bayer, 2000).

Effects and Costs

A significant problem related to ASPD is breaking the law. Some surveys
of prison populations found the rate of ASPD to be as high as 60 percent
for both men and women (Wood, 2010). Other estimates indicated that
approximately 20 percent of male and female prisoners are sociopaths,
and these prisoners are responsible for more than 50 percent of all serious crimes. Recidivism among these offenders is about double that of
other offenders and triple for violent crimes (Hare, 1993; McGregor &
McGregor, 2014).

Other estimates suggested that approximately 1 million psychopaths
are imprisoned, on parole, or on probation (Kiehl & Hoffman, 2011),
accounting for about half of all serious crimes (Hare, 1993; Haycock,
2014). Cost estimates for their crimes, trials, and confinement range
between $250 and $400 billion each year (Haycock, 2014; Kiehl &
Buckholtz, 2010).

In addition, many people with antisocial personality types commit
economic crimes that do not catch the law's attention but negatively
affect many people's lives (Dobbert, 2007).

No cost estimates are available on the pain, disappointment, and
heartbreak individuals with ASPD inflict on those around them—their
parents, spouses, children, friends, and others they interact with—but
without doubt, they are significant.

Considering a different aspect of the disorder, people with ASPD are
at a higher risk of dying from unnatural causes. People with this type of
impairment are almost four times "as likely to die violently (e.g., suicide,
accidents, and murder) as other people, according to a long-term study
(Wood, 2010).

Also, the comorbidity for ASPD with other impairments, such as pho-
bias, post-traumatic stress disorder, panic disorder, generalized anxiety
disorder, depression, and bipolar disorder, and the co-occurrence of alcohol and drug use or gambling addiction increase the sufferer's difficulties
(Wood, 2010).

On yet another level, scientists, in their search for answers, are
attempting to differentiate the working of the brains of psychopathic
and of normal people. Such research requires the use of functional

magnetic resonance imaging (fMRI) technique, which is the equivalent of a multimillion-dollar investment (Haycock, 2014).

In Society

Individuals with ASPD don't just violate social norms, such as smoking in smoking-restricted areas; they perform a variety of behaviors that constitute significant violations of the criminal code. They shoplift, break and enter households, assault with weapons, steal automobiles, and commit murder. And there are also a significant number of persons with ASPD who commit economic crimes that affect and destroy the financial lives of millions of people (Dobbert, 2007). All levels and aspects of society present a hunting ground for those who take without a thought to the damage they inflict on society. The salient feature of the criminal behaviors performed by antisocial individuals is not necessarily the violence of the behavior but the blatant disregard for others (Dobbert, 2007).

Holding others in such disregard translates in the minds of people with ASPD that it does not matter how often or how much the rights of these others are violated because they are not important enough to count for anything other than what they can give to (or be stolen from by) the antisocial perpetrator. But the level or grade of unimportance is not necessarily the same for all others in the minds of some antisocial or psychopathic individuals. People belonging to the same group as the person afflicted with ASPD may occupy a slightly more elevated position within the level of importance than the ordinary citizens outside the group.

A relevant example can be seen in the existence of different cults. Various estimates of the number of cults in the United States range from approximately 500 to 600 (*Encyclopedic Handbook of Cults in America*) to about 2,500 (Simon, 1996). Most cults have charismatic leaders, but this is not true for all cults. In general, cults are extensions of their leaders' personalities and teachings. The grandeur of a particular leader provides cult members with an essential feeling of specialness and a sense of importance. A member's relationship with the leader signifies the particular member's position or standing within the cult.

Up Close
Ambrose Sutton, a 31-year-old Caucasian male, incarcerated in the county jail, faced the forensic psychiatrist in an interview for the purpose of determining if Ambrose was competent to stand trial. Ambrose was charged with several counts of failing to register as a sexual offender.

He had been convicted of sexual misconduct with a minor. In response to the charge, Ambrose insisted that he had visited the sheriff's department in due time after his move to register but there was nobody there to help him.

While incarcerated, Ambrose informed officers he had committed a murder; he had stabbed Steve, an African American man, who had called him a child molester. Adding to Ambrose's anger was the fact that the man had been accompanied by a white girl.

Ambrose stated he had been under the influence of alcohol and felt remorse for killing the "wrong man." He later commented that this was not his first murder; admitting membership in a cult-like group, he spoke openly about his duties in the brotherhood and about those who ranked above him in the organization. It seems that Ambrose's remorse was not so much for killing someone but rather for killing the wrong *person.*

The defendant's history revealed sexual abuse suffered while growing up in a close-knit Caucasian Catholic rural community and significant chemical dependency of long standing. He graduated high school, entered into a brief marriage, and fathered five children with different partners. His criminal record listed about 10 arrests, most of them for violent acts against others. While incarcerated, he earned a bachelor of science degree.

He demonstrated angry and irritable mood, poor judgment, elated affect, rigid racial beliefs, and a tendency to blame others for his behavior. He denied current suicidal or homicidal ideation as well as hallucinations. Current mental status was alert and oriented to person, time, and place; he was deemed competent to stand trial (Mueller, 2016).

At Work

In addition to the primary diagnostic features of a pervasive disregard for the rights of others, additional features of antisocial personality disorder include irresponsible work behavior and financial irresponsibility. In work situations, individuals' antisocial behavior may be expressed in repeated absences from work that are not illness related. Furthermore, they may tend to borrow money from coworkers without repaying their debts.

Frequently, in individuals with ASPD, their contempt for the rights and feelings of others is paired with an inflated and arrogant appraisal of themselves. They may regard themselves as too smart or too important to perform ordinary work activities. Grounded in their opinions, these individuals' behaviors may come across as excessively opinionated and self-assured, or even cocky, contributing to a negative work atmosphere.

However, this inflated self-appraisal—when paired with glib, superficial charm and verbal facility—may impress a supervisor who is less verbally communicative, thus leading to undeserved promotions.

It is doubtful that persons with antisocial or psychopathic personality traits would be successful in highly structured work situations because rules and regulations mean nothing to them and the company's future goals and objectives are of little interest to them. However, they may be able—at least for a period of time—to function within a given employment situation. One researcher described a work situation in which an individual evoked contrasting opinions about him in his coworkers. While one group regarded him as the primary cause for difficulties within their department, another group considered him to be a creative and innovative individual who contributed to the company's objectives and showed true leadership characteristics (Babiak & Hare, 2006).

Obviously, the negative opinions were expressed by the members of the team he had been assigned to work with. Apparently, a review of the individual's record by the company's personnel department showed that the individual had lied on his application papers and did not possess the required education and experience that he had claimed. Furthermore, there had been incidents when he had removed company equipment for his personal use.

As the various antisocial personality traits find expression in persons afflicted with this disorder, it is not difficult to recognize their potential for negatively affecting the persons' work situations as they interact with colleagues and coworkers. The result is often dismissal or job termination. But due to these individuals' inflated self-appraisals and lack of insight into their own shortcomings, any reason for termination will be interpreted as undue and unjustified punishment, possibly even as an act of persecution. In the minds of some antisocial persons, the loss of a job may require revenge and/or acts of violence.

Up Close
Jennifer, a lively, attractive woman in her early forties, interviewed new applicants for several open positions in the special programming department of a midsized information technology firm. In her position as assistant to the director of the department, she was not actually in a position to hire anybody; instead, she was interviewing the first round of applicants in a group of possible candidates, who would be narrowed down into the "probable" individuals to be interviewed by Martin, the director. In her interviews with the applicants, after inquiries concerning the candidates' professional experience and qualifications, Jennifer—without

verbalizing it—managed to leave most of the candidates with the impression that she would recommend them for the job. So whoever was hired by Martin would believe that it was due to Jennifer's recommendation of him or her, thus ensuring the new employee's loyalty to Jennifer, who had her eyes set on Martin's position. Her marriage had ended in divorce when her husband found out that she had an affair with her boss. That's when she lost both her husband and her job—because her married boss could not afford to keep her around the office anymore. Jennifer played the victim by turning the story around, making her husband the unfaithful spouse as she reinvented her life.

Martin, unaware of Jennifer's way of handling the preselection process, hired three of the applicants. He trusted Jennifer's open, friendly demeanor and her eagerness to take on tasks that were not part of her job description. Jennifer used those tasks to spread conflicting information about the work procedures among employees, which gave Martin the appearance of a contradictive and indecisive person, ill-suited for his job. Establishing the newly hired employees' loyalty to Jennifer had not been a wasted effort.

In Relationships

Sociopathy is not just the absence of conscience, which by itself would be tragic enough; it is the inability to process emotional experiences, including those of love and caring, except when such experiences can be calculated as a coldly intellectual task. Furthermore, having a conscience is more than merely experiencing the presence of guilt and remorse; it is based in our capacity to experience emotion and the attachments that result from our feelings. At its very essence, sociopathy is ice-cold, like a dispassionate game of chess. Sociopaths cannot genuinely fall in love, but an intelligent sociopath with practice may become convincingly fluent in "conversational emotion" (Stout, 2005).

In analyzing interactive behaviors of people with ASPD, or sociopaths, with other people, observers have pointed to the existence of what they called the "Sociopath-Empath-Apath Triad (SEAT)," explaining that in order to be successful in their schemes, antisocial individuals often enlist the assistance of hangers-on. This means that the interactions involve a third party, the "apath,"—who colludes in the scheme "apathetically"—in addition to the sociopath and the target person (McGregor & McGregor, 2014).

Being apathetic within this framework means that the apath shows a lack of concern for, or is indifferent to, the targeted person. However, a main requirement for an apath is that he or she has some connection to the sociopath's target. Friends, siblings, parents, and other relations of the targets can become accomplices to the sociopath, assisting in the damage done to the target person. Whatever the reasons for the apath's involvement might be, his or her conscience seems to go to sleep during the course of interacting with the sociopath, like some people blindly follow a leader whose only motivation is one of self-interest. This type of behavior was demonstrated in experiments in the early 1960s at Yale University by professor Stanley Milgram. In the study subjects became confederates of the experimenter in engaging in seemingly harmful behaviors to others in order to please their perceived superiors (McGregor & McGregor, 2014).

"Empaths" are persons frequently targeted by individuals with ASPD. While most humans are able to empathize, some have a greater ability than others. Certain regions of their brains, the anterior cingulated cortex and anterior insula, light up in bright orange color on an fMRI scan when they witness another human being in pain (Gibson, 2006). Empaths are highly perceptive and insightful people, belonging to the estimated 40 percent of human beings who are able to detect when something is not right. They are often mediators and peacemakers. As they are sensitive to others' emotional distress, they often have difficulty comprehending that some people may lack compassion for others (McGregor & McGregor, 2014). This mental-emotional combination turns empaths into perfect targets for sociopaths, although the empath's ability to sense that something is wrong might pose a threat to the sociopath. However, this possible threat may be considered by the sociopath as an interesting challenge in an otherwise boring situation.

Whether through a triadic or any other type of interaction, antisocial individuals, with their calculated attention and affection, can initially overwhelm anybody, and their first step in any seduction is to make themselves appealing to their targets (Anderson, 2012).

Up Close

At the Starbucks café, Sandra wondered if the stranger who had contacted her through the internet dating service would recognize her. No pictures had been exchanged. Then she heard a voice saying, "You must be Sandra; you are just like in my dream!" The voice belonged to a good-looking man in his 30s who entered the restaurant, heading straight for Sandra's table. The certainty in his voice bestowed an aura of destiny to the situation. Little did Sandra know that he had been watching outside for some time. Surprised, Sandra nodded her head. He sat down and leaned across the table, his eyes never leaving her face as he said, "I am Robert; I can't wait to know more about you."

It was a whirlwind romance. Robert insisted on seeing Sandra daily— any day without her would be a lost day, he said. Robert told Sandra that he was divorcing his wife, who had made his life miserable. Until now he stayed in the marriage because of their two children. Currently he sought refuge with a friend because his ex-wife had moved all the money from their joint bank account into a secret individual account just before the divorce. Robert was heartbroken because he could not have visitation with his children in his current situation. Sandra, although disappointed about dating an almost divorced man, could not help empathizing with his sad situation and being impressed by Robert's devotion to his children.

After meeting Robert's friend, who corroborated Robert's story, Sandra let Robert move into her two-bedroom condominium, providing space for visitation with his children—after all, Robert wanted to get married as soon as the divorce was final. Before that, Robert needed money to replace some of his clothes and personal items—things his wife had destroyed in a fit of anger.

Six months into the relationship, Robert stayed away some nights. As he explained, sometimes he stayed with his friend because from there, he could walk the children home after being with them; or he stayed with the children in their home, taking care of them during his ex-wife's absence. Robert always apologized and promised to try other solutions. In the end Sandra learned that there had been no divorce, and Robert did not return to his wife; as he told Sandra when he finally left, he had found another target.

Theory and Research

Explorations of associations with ASPD have focused on comparisons of identical and nonidentical (fraternal) twins and on adoption studies. As mentioned earlier, twin studies, meant to discern between genetic and environmental effects, have reported significant genetic influences on antisocial behavior (Baker et al., 2006). Theoretically, nonidentical twins share only half of their genes, so a completely genetic disorder could be found in both twins about 50 percent of the time, whereas its concordance rate in identical twins would be close to 100 percent. Combined results of twin studies of antisocial behavior have shown concordance rates of 67 percent in identical twins and 31 percent in nonidentical twins, thus supporting genetic theories of causation (Brennan & Mednick, 1993).

A major longitudinal study investigated sociopathic traits and their absence in 3,226 pairs of male twins who had served in the United States armed services during the Vietnam War. Eight sociopathic symptoms and their absence were found to be heritable (Stout, 2005).

Adoption studies show that, in general, biological children of criminal or antisocial parents are more likely than other children to engage in criminal behavior as adults, even when early adoption removes them from the influence of their biological parents, as was found by following 52 adoptees born to 41 female criminals. Six of the adoptees—or 13 percent—were diagnosed as antisocial, compared to only 2 percent of control adoptees (Crowe, 1974).

Similar signs of genetic influence were observed in a longitudinal study (Texas Adoption Project), progressing for more than 30 years, comparing over 500 now-grown adopted children with both their biological and adopted parents. The study focused on the acquisition of intelligence and several personality features, including scores of psychopathic deviance obtained on the Minnesota Multiphasic Personality Inventory's "Psychopathic Deviate" (Pd) scale, indicated that individuals resemble their birth mothers, whom they have never met, significantly more than they do the adoptive parents who raised them. A hereditability estimate of 54 percent could be derived from the Pd score, which is consistent with the hereditability estimates—35 to 50 percent—found in other studies (Stout, 2005).

One gene of particular interest regarding antisocial behavior is the gene that encodes for monoamine oxidase A (MAO-A), an enzyme that breaks down monoamine neurotransmitters such as serotonin and norepinephrine. Studies examining the gene's relationship to behavior have indicated that variants of the gene that account for reduced MAO-A production have associations with aggressive behavior (Guo et al., May 2008; Guo et al., August 2008). Another association was found in some children whose early life included negative experiences or maltreatment and who possessed a low-activity variant (MAO-L). These children were more likely to develop antisocial behavior than those with high-activity variants (MAO-H; [Caspi et al., 2002; Frazzetto et al., 2007]). Other studies have also found a relationship between MAO-A and antisocial behavior in maltreated children (Huizinga et al., October 2006).

A meta-analysis of 20 studies indicated significantly lower serotonin levels among individuals younger than 30 years of age (Moore et al., 2002). Considering that antisocial behaviors spike during people's teenage years and decline in their 30s, the meta-analysis findings may indicate a correlation.

Within the brain, altered functioning in the cerebral cortex can bring about changes in the neurobiological-behavioral links. Studies of how human beings process language have discovered important information about cortical functioning in sociopathy. Observations of tiny electrical reactions, called "evoked potentials," at the level of electrical activity in the brain show that normal people react to emotional words, such as *love*, *hate*, or *mother*, more rapidly and more intensely than to relatively neutral words, such as *table*, *chair*, *later*, and so on. Comparing sociopaths and normal subjects in the language processing tasks demonstrated that—contrary to normal subjects—sociopathic subjects' reaction times and evoked potentials in the cortex showed no difference between emotionally charged and neutral words (Stout, 2005).

Related research with single-photon emission-computed tomography demonstrated that, compared to normal subjects, sociopathic subjects showed increased blood flow to the temporal lobes when they responded to a decision task that involved emotional words. Assignments based on emotional words, tasks that would be almost neurologically instantaneous for normal people, elicited physiological reactions in the sociopaths as if they had been requested to work out difficult problems (Stout, 2005).

Studies like those described indicate that in sociopathic individuals, an altered processing of emotional stimuli occurs at the level of the cerebral cortex (Stout, 2005).

Besides genetic and physiological influences, researchers have linked physical head injuries with antisocial behavior. An often-cited example is the case of Phineas Gage, a construction foreman who, in 1848, was injured in a quarry accident in Cavendish, Vermont. During an accidental explosion, a 13-pound iron rod was driven through his skull. Miraculously, Gage survived the accident, but his personality changed from a responsible, industrious citizen to a fitful, irreverent man, obstinate and impatient of restraint or advice. MRI technology was used with Gage's preserved skull to create computer images of his brain, showing both the location and the extent of the damage (Damasio et al., 1994).

Brain injury, including damage to the prefrontal cortex and reduction of gray matter volume in the frontal cortex, has been associated with inability to make morally and socially acceptable decisions. In addition, damage to the amygdala may interfere with the prefrontal cortex's ability to interpret feedback from the limbic system, which could result in uninhibited signals manifested in violent and aggressive behavior (Franklin Institute, 2004). The association between activity in the prefrontal cortex and antisocial behavior can now be made more apparent through functional neuroimaging as opposed to the structural neuroimaging techniques used earlier (Yang et al., 2009).

One of the associated features supporting a diagnosis of antisocial personality is the individual's lack of empathy. Some researchers theorize that the level of empathy most people experience varies according to the conditions they face at any given moment. They also assume that people's empathy level is predetermined along the "empathy spectrum," to which they return from any change. The range of the empathy spectrum is thought to go from six degrees at one end to zero degrees at the other end. Six degrees marks the location for highly empathic individuals, while sociopaths are located at zero degrees. An empathy quotient (EQ) test, developed for this research, measures how easily individuals pick up on and how strongly they are affected by others' feelings (Baron-Cohen, 2011)

These empathy changes are thought to occur deep in the human brain within a so-called "empathy circuit," which involves at least 10 interconnected brain regions. The functioning of this circuit is believed to determine where individuals lie on the empathy spectrum. This idea is related to the earlier work of Giacomo Rizzolatti, an Italian neurophysiologist, demonstrating the existence of a system of nerve cells that he called "mirror neurons," suggesting that empathy involves some form of mirroring of other people's actions and emotions (Baron-Cohen, 2011) With the use of fMRI, scientists have identified the regions of the brain that appear to be involved in the mirror neuron system (Keysers, 2011).

The consideration of psychopathy as an extension of ASPD, identifying one form of pathology associated with high levels of antisocial behavior in individuals with a particular form of emotional impairment (Blair, Mitchell, & Blair, 2005), requires the inclusion of research about this particular pathology. It has been estimated that there are over 29 million psychopaths worldwide, and one in four maximum security inmates is a psychopath (Kiehl, 2014). An urgent need for the understanding of this disorder has been voiced by some (Blair et al., 2005).

From the characteristics described in Hervey Cleckley's *Mask of Sanity* and his own clinical observations, Robert Hare developed the original Psychopathy Checklist (PCL), a tool for the assessment of psychopathy in adults, in 1986, to be followed in 1991 by the revised edition Psychopathy Checklist-Revised (PCL-R). Proponents of the concept of psychopathy emphasize the PCL-R's main advantage over the psychiatric diagnoses of conduct disorder (CD) and ASPD in that it not only indexes the individuals' behavior but also their personalities (Cleckley, 1941; Hare, 1991).

One of the urban myths regarding psychopathic individuals states that they are of above-average intellect; however, little correlation was found between IQ (using the Wechsler Adult Intelligence Scale) and both total scores on the PLC-R and emotional dysfunction scores. A modest negative correlation with antisocial behavior scores was obtained (Hare, 1991); that is, higher levels of antisocial behavior were associated with lower IQ. In fact, IQ, age, and socioeconomic status (SES) were all found to be inversely related to antisocial behavior (Hare, 2003).

According to studies, certain regions in the brains of psychopaths show less thickness in cortical density than in nonpsychopaths. This part of the brain, the temporal pole in the temporal lobe, is involved—along with other regions—in processing and recognizing emotions Furthermore, evidence of structural brain difference was found between persistently violent men with and without psychopathy. Offenders with ASPD displayed significantly reduced gray matter volumes bilaterally in the anterior rostral prefrontal cortex and temporal poles. This knowledge is thought to facilitate research into the etiology of persistent violent behavior (Gregory, 2012).

In 2000, with the use of structural MRI techniques, researchers found an 11 percent decrease in prefrontal gray matter in the brains of 21 men who had average Hare psychopathy scores of 29 out of 40. It was suggested that this prefrontal lobe deficit may be the reason for the low arousal, poor fear conditioning, lack of conscience, and deficits in decision making that characterize psychopathic behavior (Raine et al., 2000). Also, thinner cerebral cortices in about half a dozen different brain regions were found in 21 psychopathic criminal inmates when compared to incarcerated nonpsychopaths (Ly, 2012; Haycock, 2014). According to psychopath experts, these observations reinforce the notion that psychopathy is a neurobiological condition (Blair, 2012; Haycock, 2014).

As impressive as these brain cell statistics are, the goal in studies using fMRI machines is to compare activity and responses in the brains of psychopaths to activity in the brains of nonpsychopaths (Haycock, 2014).

The first to apply fMRI technology in the study of psychopathy were German scientists at the University of Düsseldorf. In their study, a dozen men between the ages of 18 and 45 years with an average PCL-R score of 29 were compared to a dozen psychologically healthy men. All 24 subjects were shown pictures of faces with neutral expressions while presenting a neutral stimulus (a puff of room air) or an aversive stimulus (a puff of rotten yeast odor). Both groups learned to associate smells with the pictures of the faces. Neither group liked the rotten smell. The fMRI images reflected the difference between the two groups as they were learning to make these associations. The psychopaths showed increased activity, while the nonpsychopaths showed decreased activity in the dorsolateral prefrontal cortex and the amygdala (brain regions closely involved in emotional responses). The increased activity in these regions observed in psychopaths was interpreted to reflect greater effort in making emotional associations between a bad smell and a particular face. It appears that the neuronal processing mechanism devoted to learning this task with an emotional component seems to be more efficient in nonpsychopaths than in psychopaths (Schneider, 2000; Haycock, 2014). Considering that the amygdala is part of the limbic region, which is weak in psychopaths, causing them to struggle in understanding emotional language, the psychopaths' difficulty with the described task would seem reasonable (Brown, 2009).

In another study made possible through the use of fMRI technology, brain scans were obtained of 16 criminals with low psychopathic traits as they reviewed images with moral connotations that were expected to evoke moral judgments. The results showed that the amygdala in the viewers' brains seemed to "light up" (experienced increased blood flow). The same results occurred when 28 noncriminals with no psychopathic traits viewed the pictures. Presentation of the same pictures to another group of 16 incarcerated men with high levels of psychopathic traits yielded considerably different results. The criminals with high psychopathic traits seemed to have *decreased* levels of activation in their amygdalae when viewing the images of moral violations (Harenski, 2010; Haycock, 2014).

Although sociopathy seems to be timeless and universal, there are differences in its occurrence in different cultures. According to information from the National Institute of Mental Health, in the 15 years preceding their study, the prevalence of ASPD had nearly doubled among the young in America. Such a rapid shift is difficult to explain in terms of genetics or neurobiology; cultural influences seem to be involved, too (Stout, 2005).

Treatment

When attempting to treat the core self and interpersonal pathology—the defining features of personality disorder—there are few empirical studies to be found, and suggestions for interventions are largely based on a conceptual analysis of the problem and what clinicians have found useful (Livesley, 2003).

ASPD is considered to be a chronic, persistent disorder that seldom remits. As a study with 524 child guidance clinic patients demonstrated, 94 were identified as antisocial in adulthood; 82 of them were interviewed in their 30s and 40s. Remission was noted for only 12 percent, showing no evidence of antisocial behavior. There had been some improvement for another 27 percent, but they were still getting into trouble. For a full 61 percent, there was no improvement at all; some were even considered worse. The median age for improvement was 35 years (Robins, 1966).

The difficulty of therapeutic interventions with ASPD is based in the characteristics of the disorder that preclude change. The consequences of the behavior—as evaluated by the patient—determine the direction of future behaviors.

In general, people with ASPD do not respond well to treatment. Group therapy may be helpful at times, especially in a residential setting. But even then, the dropout rate tends to be high. Cases of involuntary therapy (forced to do so by the courts or family members) hold an even smaller chance of success. Medication is useful primarily in reducing associated symptoms like anxiety and depression and in controlling the most violent outbursts of anger.

With increasing age, at least the most extreme manifestations of the disorder begin to subside. Usually after age 40, criminal offenses become markedly less common (Bayer, 2000).

Because there are no standard treatments for ASPD, it is essential to identify coexisting problems that *can* respond to intervention. Treating coexisting disorders can help reduce some antisocial behaviors and prepare the person for the more complicated task of addressing ASPD (Black, 2013).

Bob Johnson, MD, a consultant psychiatrist and cofounder of the James Naylor Foundation, a charity devoted to the understanding and support of those diagnosed with personality disorder in England, rejects the idea of untreatability as appalling (Johnson, 2000). Interestingly, while Johnson worked at the Parkhurst Prison, treating those considered to have Dangerous Severe Personality Disorder, the number of violent incidents decreased from 52 during the first seven years to one episode of violence in the last two years (Johnson, 1999). It is conceivable that the category of dangerous severe personality disorder included those who were antisocial personality disordered, sociopaths, and psychopaths—although detailed statistics don't seem to be available.

References

Anderson, D. (2012). *Red flags of love fraud: 10 signs you're dating a sociopath*. Egg Harbor Township, NJ: Anderly Publishing.

Babiak, P., & Hare, R. D. (2006). *Snakes in suits: When psychopaths go to work*. New York, NY: Regan Books (Imprint of HarperCollins Publishers).

Baker, L. A., Bezdjian, S., & Raine, A. (2006). Behavioral genetics: The science of antisocial behavior. *Law and Contemporary Problems, 69* (1–2), 746.

Baron-Cohen, S. (2011). *Zero degrees of empathy: A new theory of human cruelty.* London: Allen Lane/Penguin Books.

Bayer, L. (2000). *Personality disorders.* Philadelphia, PA: Chelsea House Publishers.

Black, D. W. (2013). *Bad boys, bad men: Confronting antisocial personality disorder (sociopathy)* (revised and updated). New York, NY: Oxford University Press.

Blair, J., Mitchell, D., & Blair, K. (2005). *The psychopath: Emotions and the brain.* Malden, MA: Blackwell Publishing.

Blair, R. J. R. (2012). Cortical thinning and functional connectivity in psychopathy. *American Journal of Psychiatry, 69*(7), 684–687.

Brennan, P. A., & Mednick, S. A. (1993). Genetic perspectives on crime. *Acta Psychiatrica Scandinavica, supplement 70,* 19–26.

Brown, Sandra L. (2009). *Women who love psychopaths* (2nd ed.). Penrose, NC: Mask Publishing.

Caspi, A., McClay, J., Moffitt, T. E., Mill, J., Martin, J., Craig, I. W., ... Poulton, R. (2002). Role of genotype in the cycle of violence in maltreated children. *Science, 297*(5582), 851–854.

Castillo, Heather. (2003). *Personality disorder—Temperament or trauma? (An account of an emancipatory research study carried out by service users diagnosed with personality disorder).* Philadelphia, PA: Jessica Kingsley Publishers (Forensic Focus 23).

Cleckley, Hervey M. (1941). *The mask of sanity.* St. Louis, MO: Mosby.

Compton, W. M., Conway, K. P., Stinson, F. S., Colliver, J. D., & Grant, B. F. (2005). Prevalence, correlates, and comorbidity of DSM-IV antisocial personality syndromes and alcohol and specific drug use disorders in the United States: Results from the National Epidemiologic Survey on Alcohol and Related Conditions. *Journal of Clinical Psychiatry, 66,* 677–685.

Craft, M. (1966). The meanings of the term psychopath. In M. Critter (Ed.), *Psychopathic disorders.* New York, NY: Pergamon Press.

Crowe, R. (1974). An adoption study of antisocial personality. *Archives of General Psychiatry, 31,* 784–791.

Damasio, H., Grabowski, T., & Frank, R. (1994). The return of Phineas Gage: Lies about the brain from the skull of a famous patient. *Science, 264,* 1112–1115.

Dobbert, D. L. (2007). *Understanding personality disorders.* Lanham, MD: Rowman & Littlefield Publishers.

The Franklin Institute to honor the 2004 Benjamin Franklin Medal and Bower Award Laureates. April 29, 2004 (PRIMEZONE), Philadelphia, PA. Retrieved from http://www.fi.edu/tfiawards

Frazzetto, G., Di Lorenzo, G., Carola, V., Proietti, L., Sokolowska, E., Siracusano, A., ... Troisi, A. (2007). Early trauma and increased risk for physical aggression during adulthood: The moderating role of MAOA genotype. *PLoS One, 2*(5), e486. HYPERLINK "https://doi.org/10.1371/journal.pone%200000486" https://doi.org/10.1371/journal.pone 0000486

Gelder, M., Gath, D., & Mayou, R. (1989). Personality disorder. In *Oxford text book of antisocial psychiatry* (2nd ed.). Oxford: Oxford Medical Publications.

Gibson, L. (2006). Mirrored emotions. *University of Chicago Magazine, 98,* 4.

Goodwin, D., & Guze, S. (1989). *Psychiatric diagnosis* (4th ed., p. 240). New York, NY: Oxford University Press.

Gregory, S., Ffytche, D., Simmons, A., Kumavi, V., Howard, M., Hodgins, S., & Blackwood, N. (2012). The antisocial brain: Psychopathy matters, a structural MRI investigation of antisocial male violent offenders. *Archives of General Psychiatry, 69*(9), 962–972.

Guo, G., Ou, X. M., Roettger, M., & Shih, J. C. (May 2008). The VNTR 2 repeat in MAOA and delinquent behavior in adolescence and young adulthood: Associations and MAOA promoter activity. *European Journal of Human Genetics, 16*(5), 626–634.

Guo, G., Roettger, M., & Shih, J. C. (August 2008). The integration of genetic propensities into social-control models of delinquency and violence among male youths. *American Sociological Review, 73*(4): 543–568.

Hare, R. D. (1991). *The Hare psychopathy checklist—Revised.* Toronto, Ontario: Multi-Health Systems.

Hare, R. D. (1993). *Without conscience: The disturbing world of the psychopaths among us* (p. 74). New York, NY: The Guilford Press.

Hare, R. D. (2003). *Manual for the revised psychopathy checklist* (2nd ed.). Toronto, Ontario: Multi-Health Systems.

Harenski, C. L., Harenski, K. A., Shane, M. S., & Kiehl, K. A. (2010). Aberrant neural processing of moral violations in criminal psychopaths. *Journal of Abnormal Psychology, 119*(4), 863–874.

Haycock, Dean A. (2014). *Murderous minds: Exploring the criminal psychopathic brain: Neurological imaging and the manifestation of evil.* New York, NY: Pegasus Books.

Huizinga, D., Haberstick, B. C., Smolen, A., Menard, S., Young, S. E., Corley, R. P., ... Hewitt, J. K. (October 2006). Childhood maltreatment, subsequent antisocial behavior, and the role of Monoamine Oxidase A genotype. *Biological Psychiatry, 60*(7), 677–683.

Johnson, R. (1999). *Is humanity born loveable, sociable and non-violent?* Paper given at the Inaugural Conference of the James Naylor Foundation, 3–18, London, April 24, 1999.

Johnson, R. (2000). *Defeating the pessimism surrounding treatment.* Paper given at the Annual Conference of the James Naylor Foundation, 40–66, London, April 29, 2000.

Keysers, C. (2011). *The empathic brain: How the understanding of mirror neurons changes our understanding of human nature.* Amsterdam: Social Brain Press.

Kiehl, K. A. (2014). *The psychopath whisperer: The science of those without conscience.* New York, NY: Crown Publishers.

Kiehl, K. A., & Buckholtz, J. W. (2010). Inside the mind of a psychopath. *Scientific American Mind*, September/October, 24.

Kiehl, K. A., & Hoffman, M. (2011). The criminal psychopath: History, neuroscience, treatment, and economics in jurimetrics. *The Journal of Law, Science & Technology, 51*(4), 355–397.

Livesley, John W. (2003). *Practical management of personality disorder.* New York, NY: The Guilford Press.

Ly, M., Motzkin, J. C., Philippi, C. L., Kirk, G. B., Newman, J. P., Kiehl, K. A., & Koenigs, M. (2012). Cortical thinning in psychopathy. *American Journal of Psychiatry, 69*(7), 743–749.

McGregor, Jane, & McGregor, Tim. (2014). *The sociopath at the breakfast table.* Alameda, CA: Hunter House Inc., Publishers.

Moore, T. M., Scarpa, A., & Raine, A. (2002). A meta-analysis of serotonin metabolite 5-IAA and antisocial behavior. *Aggressive Behavior, 28*(4), 299–316.

Mueller, R., (2016). *Psychiatric evaluation.* Allen County Superior Court, IN.

Raine, A., Lencz, T., Bihrle, S., & LaCasse, L. (2000). Reduced prefrontal gray matter volume and reduced autonomic activity in antisocial personality disorder. *Archives of General Psychiatry, 57*(2), 119–127.

Robins, L. N. (1966). *Deviant children grow up.* Baltimore, MD: Williams & Wilkins.

Schneider, F., Kessler, C., Grodd, W., Habel, U., Posse, S., & Mueller-Gaertner, H. W. (2000). Functional imaging of conditioned aversive emotional responses in antisocial personality disorder. *Neuropsychobiology, 42*(4), 192–201.

Simon, Robert I. (1996). *Bad men do what good men dream.* Washington, D.C.: American Psychiatric Press.

Stout, Martha. (2005). *The sociopath next door: The ruthless versus the rest of us.* New York, NY: Harmony Books (imprint of Crown Publishing Group).

Wood, Jeffrey C. (2010). *The cognitive behavioral therapy workbook for personality disorders.* Oakland, CA: New Harbinger Publications.

Yang, Y., Raine, A., Narr, K. I., Colletti, P., & Toga, A. W. (2009). Localization of deformations within the amygdalae of individuals with pychopathy. *Archives of General Psychiatry, 66,* 986–994.

CHAPTER 2

Avoidant Personality Disorder

Symptoms, Diagnosis, and Incidence

Essential features of this disorder, which falls into cluster C, are a pervasive pattern of social inhibition, feelings of inadequacy, and hypersensitivity to negative evaluations by others. This hypersensitivity starts in early adulthood and is expressed in a variety of contexts. Because of their fears of criticism or disapproval, individuals suffering from the disorder tend to avoid work situations that involve much interpersonal contact. The feared criticism, disapproval, or rejection is generally assumed and expected by people with avoidant personality disorder, which means that anyone wanting closer contact with the person has to prove his or her acceptance or support before the avoidant person will be open to being approached. Unless they receive repeated offers of support and nurturance, individuals with avoidant personality disorder will refrain from joining group activities, or—if they have to attend group activities—they will remain mentally and emotionally distant for fear of being ridiculed or shamed.

For the same reasons, people with avoidant personality disorder shy away from new experiences because there is always the risk that they will not know how to behave and thus encounter criticism. Potential dangers of being exposed are exaggerated to the point of certainty of rejection. Somatic symptoms may serve as reasons for avoiding new activities or new situations.

The combination of low self-esteem and hypersensitivity to rejection leads to an isolated life for those afflicted with this disorder. Furthermore, depression and anxiety are often diagnosed in conjunction with avoidant personality disorder.

Other personality disorders, such as paranoid, schizoid, or schizotypal personality disorder and at times borderline personality disorder, tend to be diagnosed with avoidant personality disorder.

Often the avoidant behavior starts in childhood, but because shyness and fear of strangers are common traits in children and expected to gradually dissipate with increasing age, this tends to be overlooked as a possible precursor of avoidant personality disorder.

Based on data from the 2001–2002 National Epidemiologic Survey on Alcohol and Related Conditions, the prevalence of avoidant personality disorder is estimated to be about 2.4 percent, and it appears to be equally frequent in males and females. Other estimates state that avoidant personality disorder is the most common personality disorder, affecting roughly 1 in every 20 Americans, whereas still other estimates suggest that approximately 1 percent of the general population is afflicted with the disorder (Wood, 2010). Still other clinical studies mention that AvPD affects between 1.8 and 6.4 percent of the general population (Out of the FOG, 2018). One study noted that AvPD was seen in 14.7 percent of psychiatric outpatients (Zimmerman, Rothschild, & Chelminski, 2005). UK Hospital Admission Statistics in 2006–2007 mentioned that 43 percent of those admitted with a diagnosis of AvPD were male, and 57 percent were female.

Avoidant personality disorder—like most personality disorders—will decrease in intensity with age, with many patients experiencing few of the most extreme symptoms by the time they reach their 40s or 50s.

As mentioned in the *DSM-5*'s alternative model for personality disorders, characteristic difficulties for AvPD individuals occur in the life categories of identity, self-direction, empathy, and/or intimacy—along with specific maladaptive traits in the domains of Negative Affectivity and Detachment.

According to the *DSM-5*, avoidant personality disorder needs to be differentiated from similar personality disorders like dependent, paranoid, schizoid, and schizotypal, even though they can also occur together. This might be especially likely to occur for AvPD and dependent personality disorder.

Another overlap can at times be found in avoidant and schizoid personality traits, and there may be a relationship between AvPD and the schizophrenia spectrum (Fogelson & Nuechterlein, 2007)—with or without post-traumatic stress disorder (PTSD) (Gratz & Tull, 2012). Substance use disorders are another impairment common in individuals with AvPD, especially the use of alcohol, benzodiazepines, and heroin

(Verheul, 2001). These substances may have a significant effect on a patient's prognosis.

Individuals with AvPD are prone to self-loathing and, in some cases, self-harm. Especially those individuals who have comorbid PTSD show the highest rates of engaging in self-harming behaviors, even more than individuals with borderline personality disorder (BPD).

In the United Kingdom, reportedly 0.8 percent of people suffer from AvPD at least once in their lives, and men are more likely than women to develop this disorder: 1.0 percent versus 0.7 percent (Coid, Yang, Tyrer, Roberts, & Ullrich, 2006).

In the World Health Organization's ICD-10, AvPD is listed as anxious (avoidant) personality disorder.

Timeline

1911 Eugen Bleuler described patients with signs of avoidant personality disorder.
1921 Kretschmer provided the first relatively complete description.

History

Avoidant personality has been described in several sources as far back as the early 1900s, but it did not receive that name until sometime later. Swiss psychiatrist Eugen Bleuler described patients who showed signs of avoidant personality disorder in his work *Dementia Praecox: Or the Group of Schizophrenias.*

Kretschmer (1921) provided the first relatively complete description of avoidant personality disorder, until then avoidant and schizoid patterns were frequently confused or referred to synonymously. In 1993, Alden and Capreol defined two other subtypes of avoidant personality disorder: the Cold-avoidant and Exploitable-avoidant types (McLean & Woody, 2001).

Psychologist Theodore Millon stated that most patients present a mixed picture of symptoms, making their personality disorder a blend of a major disorder type with one or more secondary personality disorder types. He identified four adult subtypes of avoidant personality disorder (Millon, 2015).

Earlier theorists proposed a personality disorder consisting of a combination of features from borderline personality disorder and avoidant personality disorder, called "avoidant-borderline mixed personality disorder" (AvPD/BPD) (Kantor, 1993/2003).

The first decade of the 21st century saw some controversy regarding the question of whether avoidant personality disorder is different from generalized anxiety disorder. The diagnostic criteria for both disorders are similar, and they may have similar causation, course, subjective experience, and treatment as well as identical personality features, such as shyness (Nedic, Zivanovic, & Lisulov, 2011). Some experts consider them to be merely different conceptualizations of the same disorder, with avoidant personality disorder representing the more severe form. Individuals with AvPD experience more severe social phobia (SP) symptoms, and their depression and functional impairment are more severe than in generalized social phobia (GSP) alone (Reich, 2009), even though they show no differences in social skills or in delivering an impromptu speech (Herbert, Hope, & Bellack, 1992). Another difference is that SP is the *fear of social circumstances*, but AvPD would be better described as an *aversion to intimacy in relationships* (Comer, 2014).

Development and Causes

The causes of AvPD are not well defined, but a combination of social, genetic, and psychological factors seems to have an influence. Most professionals subscribe to a biopsychosocial model of causation, including the ways individuals interact with others during their early development, how their personality and temperament are shaped by their environment, and the coping skills they have learned to deal with stress and setbacks. There also may be a connection to inherited temperamental factors (Sutherland, 2006), which may provide the individual with a genetic predisposition toward AvPD (Lenzenweger & Clarkin, 2005).

While some research indicated a heritability of 0.61, there is also a strong connection between childhood abuse (sexual, physical, and emotional) and the development of AvPD (Barends Psychology, 2018). Parental behaviors, such as low parental affection or nurturing, are thought to be associated with an elevated risk of AvPD, which was noted when these children reached adulthood. Childhood emotional abuse was reported by 61 percent of adults with AvPD.

Other research indicates that a combination of high sensory processing sensitivity coupled with adverse childhood experiences may increase the risk of an individual developing AvPD (Meyer, Ajchenbrenner, & Bowles, 2005).

Apparently, a history of trauma is present in 75.8 percent of people afflicted with AvPD, and 37.1 percent of those have lifetime PTSD. Furthermore, unwanted sexual contact (34.2%), followed by having a serious accident (31.4%) and witnessing injury/killing (29.4%) are some of the most reported traumatic experiences in people with AvPD. Childhood sexual abuse was experienced by 22.2 percent of individuals with AvPD, and 23.1 percent experienced childhood sexual assault (Barends Psychology, 2018).

Individuals' avoidant behavior often starts in childhood, or even infancy, with shyness, isolation, and fear of strangers and new situations. In contrast to the childhood shyness that, in most individuals, tends to gradually dissipate with increasing age, those individuals who develop AvPD experience increased shyness and avoidance during their adolescence and early adulthood, when social relationships with new people become especially important. Both childhood emotional neglect (particularly rejection by a parent) and peer group rejection are associated with an increased risk for the development of the disorder. However, it is also possible for AvPD to occur without abuse or neglect histories. Examinations of adults with AvPD indicate that those adults who experienced positive achievements and interpersonal relationships during childhood and adolescence were more likely to remit from AvPD as adults (Rettew, 2008).

Some scientists claim that the exact causes for avoidant personality disorder are unknown (Sederer, 2009); others have observed that parents of avoidant children seemed to have been troubled by their own negative emotions (Connors, 1997).

Twin studies have found that 35 percent genetic effect is accounting for avoidant personality disorder, while the majority (83%) of these genes are also linked to other personality disorders.

Effects and Costs

This disorder leaves its sufferers with an overwhelming and life-interfering feeling of not being good enough, fearing that others will view them negatively, and of being extremely shy and worried about rejection (Salters-Pedneault, 2017). Individuals with AvPD have a tendency to catastrophize, automatically assuming a "worst-case scenario" and inappropriately characterizing minor or moderate problems as catastrophic events. This tendency will lead them to withdraw from many life events and activities, at times including maintaining adequate employment. This may, in turn, cause them to require public assistance for their personal needs. This pattern, combined with the individuals' conformation bias (a tendency to pay more attention to things that reinforce their beliefs rather than to things that contradict them), leaves them unable to conceive of any beneficial change.

Avoidant personality disorder is a poorly studied personality disorder; considering prevalence rates, societal costs, and the current state of research, it qualifies as a neglected disorder (Weinbrecht, 2016).

In Society

The main difficulties associated with this disorder occur in social and occupational functioning. People with AvPD generally believe that they are unwelcome in social situations, regardless of whether such beliefs have any basis in reality. The low self-esteem and hypersensitivity to rejection lead to significantly restricted interpersonal contacts. Unless they are certain that they will be liked and accepted, most people with AvPD see themselves as socially inept or personally unappealing. They avoid social interaction for fear of being ridiculed, humiliated, or rejected, even though they very much desire to belong.

When they can't avoid social situations, they will not speak up for fear of saying the wrong thing, or blushing, or stammering, and anxiously watching those around them for signs of approval or rejection. They will stay on the periphery of the interaction, giving only monosyllable answers to direct questions. And they are especially afraid of teasing; even good-natured teasing will make them feel extremely uncomfortable.

The possibility of social rejection is so painful that persons with AvPD will choose to be alone rather than risk trying to connect with others and be shunned. Many of these people view themselves with contempt (Millon & Davis, 1996). They cannot imagine possessing any traits that are generally considered as positive within their societies.

It has been noted that people with avoidant personality disorder may be so afraid of criticism that they refuse to leave their home. They might even remove themselves from society to live far from human contact.

Up Close
Nancy's childhood years were spent as a single, painfully shy, and quiet child, afraid of strangers and almost equally afraid of neighbors because they might tease her. Nancy stayed close to her mother, a quiet unassuming woman who did not entertain or visit friends. Neither Nancy nor her mother seemed to be close to Nancy's father, who traveled a lot on business. His presence at home was that of a visitor rather than

a family member. Nancy's parents did not seem to share an atmosphere of intimacy. Much later Nancy learned that her father had been involved in various sexual relationships while on business travel.

During her school years, Nancy tried to remain unnoticed by most of her classmates as well as by her teachers. Although intelligent enough, she did not excel in anything, believing that she was not as smart as any of her classmates. Most of her school time was spent in a high state of anxiety, fearing that a teacher might call on her and she would not have the answer. She never dated any of the boys in her classes and, as would be expected, did not attend her high school prom. She graduated from high school as quietly as she had attended.

High school graduation presented a problem: What was Nancy going to do for her future life? She did not have the courage to move to a college away from home, yet she had to become responsible for her own adult life at some point. During her lonely school years, Nancy had developed an interest in nature and usually took walks by herself, exploring woods and parks within their county. She was a frequent visitor at the local library and read many books on biology and botany.

A community college seemed to be the solution. She could still live at home and attend classes almost as unobserved as she had done during her school years. Continuing with her interest in botany and biology, she was able to connect with training leading to employment within the national park–ranger system. Within that environment Nancy led a solitary life, shared only by her dog and two cats.

At Work

The person with AvPD would rather not go to work because in most work settings, he or she will be confronted by other people and by some required interaction with them.

The general sense of inhibition, inadequacy, and hypersensitivity to criticism that individuals with AvPD are plagued with may induce them to withdraw from work or school activities for fear of rejection. It is not difficult to understand that such behaviors will not be acceptable in many workplaces and may lead to repeated terminations if the person has not already left of his or her own accord. In addition, they may pass up opportunities for occupational advancement for fear that such advancement would confront them with new responsibilities. As they exaggerate any possible dangers in unknown situations, they are likely to cancel a job interview, claiming a cold or headache as excuse to avoid what seems dangerous or possibly embarrassing to them.

The avoidant behaviors of individuals with AvPD can also adversely affect their occupational functioning because they tend to avoid not only any teamwork—work activities that involve contact with others for fear of criticism, disapproval, or rejection—but also the types of social situations that may be important for meeting the basic demands of the job or for job advancement (Bressert, 2017).

Always fearful of possible criticism, individuals with AvPD tend to avoid or even reject luncheon gatherings with colleagues, thereby earning the reputation of being arrogant and unfriendly. The social frivolities of office colleagues is viewed by the afflicted person as terrifying because the afflicted person fears to become the target of teasing (Dobbert, 2007).

Up Close

At the age of 51, Donald was at the end of his career, although, financially, he could not afford to quit working. Donald's vision problems disqualified him from continuing his work as a subway driver. But that was all he knew. As a child, growing up in a big city, he had been a disappointment to his father, who wanted his only son to be athletic—he should join his high school football team or at least be on the running or any other kind of athletic team. Donald's one-year-younger sister, Annette, was already on the swim team. Donald, however, did not seem interested in any sport. He was a shy, timid boy, with no friends. The other children often made fun of him because it was so easy to embarrass him. In class, he hardly ever raised his hand to volunteer an answer to one of the teacher's questions—even if he knew the answer. What was worse, when the teacher called on him, Donald stumbled over his words, unable to give a coherent answer. Donald did not have a speech impediment; it was the unbearably strong anxiety that prevented him from communicating effectively.

Donald had no place to hide. In school he was at the mercy of his classmates—some of them bullied him, and others teased him—and at home, his father left no doubt that he was ashamed of his son. His mother felt sorry for Donald and tried to cheer him up by giving him special treats like candy, cookies, and little ice-cream surprises. His mother meant well, but the increased weight made Donald look like a big sponge and, of course, resulted in more teasing.

Because school was a nightmare for Donald, he was not interested in improving his skills in the subjects of his classes. But he did develop an interest in trains and automobiles. It was not so much the manufacturing side of these modes of transportation as the actual driving. In his mind, it seemed that by driving, he could outrun the fear, confusion, and anxiety within himself because he could flee from any painful and punishing interaction with others. At some point Donald considered becoming a delivery driver or perhaps a bus driver, but both occupations still involved too much interaction with the public. Donald was suspicious of everybody. Driving a subway train seemed the safest thing to do. He could see himself driving pretty much the same route day by day, except for occasionally having to fill in for another driver. Face-to-face contact with the public was at a minimum; all he had to worry about were his supervisors and brief contacts with other drivers. Not much change would occur in this occupation, which eliminated another reason for anxiety.

Probably the biggest change in Donald's life came when he married Susan, a quiet girl from his high school. Although they had some things in common, such as shyness and low self-esteem, that did not help in forming secure, close bonds with each other. Donald's extreme sensitivity to negative evaluations from others kept him from opening up and attempting emotional intimacy with Susan. After some time they became the parents of a little girl, which provided Susan with an object for her love. As the marriage disintegrated, Susan left with their little daughter, leaving Donald by himself. He did not appear uncomfortable with his now solitary life and never dated another woman.

Now Donald had lost not only his family but also, to him, an even bigger loss: his job. Medical opinion did not pronounce the eye impairment sufficiently severe to render Donald eligible for disability payments from the government or his insurance. Finding a new source of income was frightening—what kind of work could he do, being afraid of changes and of people? Thoughts of suicide entered his mind.

In Relationships

If they manage to be in relationships, individuals with AvPD can be overly critical as a defense mechanism, ultimately ending up alienating a friend or spouse. Within intimate relationships they exhibit restraint because of their fear of being shamed or ridiculed. As they have little interest in sexual activities and experience little pleasure from sensory, bodily, or erotic activity, they usually don't date or marry. Yet, they do desire affection and acceptance and may fantasize about ideal relationships rather than actually engage in them (Bayer, 2000). They may fantasize about idealized, accepting, and affectionate relationships because of their desire to belong. But, feeling unworthy of the relationships they desire, individuals with the disorder shame themselves from ever attempting to begin them (Hoeksema, 2014).

Individuals with AvPD may be afraid to share personal information or talk about their feelings, which makes it difficult to maintain intimate relationships. Deep down the afflicted person has trouble believing that anyone is really going to like him or her. Those who suffer from AvPD may use withdrawal as a form of communicating or as a way of emotional control over friends, partners, and family members.

As romantic relationships generally become less formal, teasing and playful comments become more prevalent between partners. But the person afflicted with AvPD does not have enough of a "sense of humor" to understand that this is part of the progression from formal to casual and then from casual to intimate behavior and, therefore, is not able to respond appropriately. This, in turn, leaves the other partner confused, often leading to termination of the relationship before it even begins to become intimate.

Romantic relationships with a person afflicted with AvPD may exert undue stress on the healthy partner because the person suffering from the disorder will try to pull the partner away from family, friends, and everyday social settings. Those in relationships with persons who suffer from AvPD may also experience pressure to isolate themselves along with the afflicted partner, or they may feel the pressure to protect them from criticism by creating an artificial or dysfunctional "bubble" or ideal environment just for the two of them, where they can escape the risk of criticism and negative self-thought.

Up Close

Twenty-nine-year-old Irene had been painfully shy all her life. Although pretty in her own way, she grew up in the shadow of her vivacious older sister, Susan. Susan was smart and popular in school, and her parents were proud of her. Irene disliked school because her teachers remembered having had Susan in their classes and tended to compare Irene to Susan—a comparison that did not come out in Irene's favor. Irene sat in the back row of her classrooms, trying to fade into the background. Although she did not like to attend school, Irene spent a lot of time on her homework. Because of the teasing—and sometimes bullying—she did not feel comfortable playing with the other children in her neighborhood. She preferred studying in the safety of her home.

In her loneliness, Irene developed a skill for writing. What she was afraid to express in the presence of others, she tried to say on paper. However, she was always in fear of criticism because she did not believe whatever she did was as good as what her classmates did. It did not help her when one day, as the teacher handed back the homework to the class, she accused Irene of having handed in a story written by Susan instead of her own work. Irene tried to defend herself in her shy, timid way but the teacher, believing Irene was not intelligent enough to have written that story, remained convinced that Irene had been cheating. Irene shied away from further confrontation with the teacher; however, the incident increased her distrust and fear of other people. She became even more withdrawn.

Following graduation from high school, Irene was able to secure employment in a big warehouse, keeping track of the various inventories. She did not have to face customers, and it did not require much interaction with coworkers. She was reluctant to take any risks or engage in new activities and never considered any opportunities for occupational advancement, because that might entail new responsibilities or new people to interact with.

Her dating history was equally uneventful. On some dates her anxiety was so strong that she could hardly speak in a coherent manner because her attention was focused on the young man's speech, trying to detect criticism or rejection. If someone did not treat her nicely, she swallowed her anger and did not complain, but as a result, she became more depressed and had difficulty sleeping. Her parents had become aware of her sleep disturbance and her depressed mood and insisted that Irene talk to their family physician, who prescribed antidepressant and antianxiety medications. When Irene's condition did not improve significantly, he referred her to a psychiatrist, who diagnosed Irene's condition as AvPD and suggested that she participate in an experimental group therapy experience to help individuals with dependent personality disorder and those with AvPD adjust to and work through the difficulties the disorders presented to them. At first Irene disliked the idea, but she was not used to putting up resistance to the requests of others, and she told herself that because the other group members experienced difficulties similar to her own, they would understand her pain and discomfort, making it a safe place for her.

Robert, one of the group members, seemed to suffer even more than Irene did. He did not show any positive emotions about anything or anybody. Irene felt sorry for him and responded positively to him when he asked her for a favor. This was the beginning of their relationship. They dated outside the group meetings and decided to get married. Their relationship was not a very romantic one, as Robert did not seem able to express tender feelings toward Irene. But, although Irene had a desire for intimacy, she did not complain and did not ask for Robert's loving attention; she swallowed her disappointment silently.

Marriage did not improve their relationship; if anything, Robert felt freer to express any disappointment or anger, blaming Irene for whatever did not work out between them. Robert turned to alcohol to deal with his disappointments in life. Alcohol consumption helped him to express his anger more freely, occasionally punctuating those expressions with a physical blow toward Irene's body. Again, Irene did not express her pain or anger at Robert, afraid to increase Robert's explosiveness. However, one Friday evening, after particularly explosive behavior, amplified by generous alcohol intake, Robert punched her to the floor, where she remained for some time because the pain she experienced made her fear that her left ankle might be broken. Robert had gone into their bedroom and apparently passed out on the bed. When she did not hear any noises other than his snoring, she crept slowly along the floor until she could reach the telephone and call 911. After her release from the hospital, Irene's parents took her home to recover from her broken ankle and her broken marriage.

Theory and Research

Depending on the characteristics of study samples, research findings regarding the co-occurrence of AvPD and BPD show different results. One study found that in their treatment sample of BPD individuals, 43 percent also met the diagnostic criteria for AvPD; and in another study, using a community sample, over 11 percent of individuals diagnosed with BPD in their lifetime also met the criteria for AvPD in their lifetime. Although the reasons for this co-occurrence are not known, experts have considered that one of the reasons for the comorbidity may be that AvPD and BPD share a key symptom—an intense fear of criticism and rejection.

Examinations of adults with avoidant personality disorder showed that childhood lack of involvement with peers and failure to engage in structured activities may continue through adolescence and adulthood in these individuals. On the other hand, adults who had positive achievement and interpersonal relationships during childhood and adolescence were more likely to remit from avoidant personality disorder as adults (Rettew, 2008).

As mentioned earlier, it has also been theorized that certain cases of AvPD may develop when individuals with innately high sensory processing sensitivity (characterized by deeper processing of physical and emotional stimuli, accompanied by high levels of empathy) are raised in abusive, negligent, or otherwise dysfunctional environments, which disturbs their ability to form secure bonds with others (Meyer et al., 2005).

In a study of patients with major depressive disorder undergoing a six-month treatment, it was found that the presence of symptoms of avoidant personality disorder was associated with poorer outcomes (Mulder, Joyce, Frampton, Luty, & Sullivan, 2006).

A study published in 2003 in the *Journal of the American Academy of Childhood and Adolescent Psychiatry* stated that adults with AvPD were less involved in hobbies, less popular, and showed poorer athletic performance than their peers during adolescence (Rettew et al., 2003). This can be understood as an example of early social withdrawal behavior by those afflicted with AvPD.

The diagnoses of AvPD and SP have evolved from different historical sources, but their criteria seemed to have converged in *DSM-III-R*. When 50 anxiety disorder clinic patients with *DSM-III-R* diagnosis of SP were evaluated for presence *of DSM-III-R* symptoms of AvPD, AvPD was found in 89 percent of those with the generalized subtype of social phobia (GSP) and in 21 percent of those with the discrete subtype of social phobia (DSP) (Schneier, Spitzer, Gibbon, Feyer, & Liebowitz, 1991).

Examining the relationship between SP subtypes and AvPD and their effects on impairment severity and outcome of cognitive behavioral treatment, it was found that previous treatment measures differentiated only between generalized and nongeneralized SP subtypes. AvPD was not predictive of treatment outcome (Brown, Heimberg, & Juster, 1995).

Regarding comorbidity, AvPD reportedly is especially prevalent in people with anxiety disorder, but estimates vary widely. According to research, approximately 10–50 percent of people who have panic disorder with agoraphobia have AvPD, as well as 20–40 percent of people with social anxiety disorder. In addition, AvPD is more prevalent in persons with comorbid social anxiety disorder and generalized anxiety disorder than in those who have only one of the aforementioned conditions. A 1955 study revealed that both panic disorder and SP were eight to nine times more likely to occur in people with AvPD. Similarly, the Collaborative Longitudinal Study of Personality Disorders, published in 2000, presented a whole list of co-occurring mental disorders with AvPD (Gunderson et al., 2000). Other studies have reported AvPD prevalence rates of up to 45 percent among people with generalized anxiety disorder and up to 56 percent among those with obsessive-compulsive disorder (Van Velzen, 2002). Another disorder that is commonly comorbid with AvPD is PTSD (Gratz & Tull, 2012).

Co-occurrence of avoidant and borderline personality disorders: The research findings regarding this co-occurrence vary in connection with the characteristics of the particular study sample. For instance, in a treatment sample of individuals with BPD, 43 percent of the BPD patients also met the diagnostic criteria for AvPD. In another study using a community sample, over 11 percent of individuals who met BPD criteria in their lifetime also met criteria for AvPD (Tomko, Trull, Wood, & Sher, 2014). The reasons for this co-occurrence are unknown, but it has been suggested that AvPD and BPD share a key symptom: both are associated with intense fear of rejection and criticism, and perhaps some people with BPD experience such intense emotional pain in their relationships that they may withdraw from relationships altogether in order to reduce the pain.

As mentioned earlier, considering the current state of research, avoidant personality disorder qualifies as a neglected disorder (Weinbrecht, 2016).

It is noteworthy that the case history described in the "Up Close" part of the "In Relationships" section above includes two individuals diagnosed with avoidant personality disorder, Irene and Robert, yet their behaviors show significant differences in some aspects. While both are tense and anxious in the presence of others and have the tendency to withdraw from interactions with others, Irene exhibits the inability to express anger, and she can't resist coercion or demands placed upon her by others. Robert did not have any difficulty expressing anger and other negative emotions; in fact, he seems incapable of experiencing and expressing positive emotions toward Irene and others. The behavioral characteristics exhibited by Irene and Robert tend to lend support to Alden and Capreol's proposal of two subtypes of AvPD mentioned earlier (McLean & Woody, 2001), with Irene presenting the proposed "exploitable-avoidant" subtype and Robert displaying the "cold-avoidant" subtype.

Although AvPD is a common chronic disorder with an early onset and lifelong impact, it is under-recognized and poorly studied. Furthermore, little is known regarding the most effective treatments. It is often viewed as a severe variant of social anxiety disorder. The focus of recent research has been on the phenomenology of AvPD factors of possible etiological significance, such as early parenting experiences, attachment style, temperament, and cognitive processing.

The existence of symptom similarity between AvPD and SP/anxiety has stimulated several studies involving and comparing both disorders. Clinical manifestations of SP were studied in a diagnosed sample of 21 individuals with social phobia (aged 21–53 years). SP was found to be a chronic and pervasive condition affecting various areas of life and producing significant emotional distress. Then, in a second study, individuals with a diagnosis of SP or AvPD were compared using a subsample of

10 socially phobic subjects and a sample of 8 subjects with AvPD (aged 30–60 years). Physiological reactivity and cognitive content were essentially the same for the two groups in a number of situational tasks, but those subjects with a diagnosis of AvPD appeared to be more sensitive interpersonally and exhibited significantly poorer social skills than the subjects with SP (Turner, Beidel, Dancu, & Keys, 1986).

Generalized and specific subtypes of SP were reliably diagnosed in a large sample of social phobics (n = 89). The generalized subtype exhibited a consistent pattern of greater symptom severity than did the specific subtype. In the same study, conducting a comparison of generalized social phobics with and without AvPD, a difference was found for only one of four parameters (Turner, Beidel, & Townsley, 1992).

In order to classify SPs by subtype and presence of avoidant personality disorder, GSPs with and without AvPD (n = 10 and 10) and nongeneralized SPs without AvPD (n = 10) were distinguished on measures of phobia severity. The generalized groups also showed earlier age at onset and higher scores on measures of depression, fear of negative evaluation, and social anxiety and avoidance than did the nongeneralized group. The group of individuals with SP and with AvPD endorsed more frequently AvPD criteria of general timidity and risk aversion than the other groups. The conclusion was that the obtained data indicated that both the generalized subtype of SP and the presence of AvPD provide useful diagnostic information, but the additional diagnosis of AvPD may simply identify a severe subgroup of SP (Holt, Heimberg, & Hope, 1992).

As disorders of pervasive social anxiety and inhibition are divided into the two categories of GSP and AvPD, a study explored the discriminative validity of this categorization by examining the comorbidity of GSP and AvPD and by comparing these groups on anxiety level, social skills, dysfunctional cognitions, impairment in functioning, and presence of concurrent disorders. The results obtained from 23 subjects showed high comorbidity of the two diagnoses. All subjects who met criteria for AvPD also met criteria for GSP. AvPD was associated with greater social anxiety, impairment in functioning, and comorbidity with other psychopathology. However, there was no difference in social skills or performance on an impromptu speech. It was concluded that GSP and AvPD seem to represent quantitatively different variants of the same spectrum of psychopathology rather than qualitatively different disorders (Herbert et al., 1992).

There are some indications in the literature on social cognition as it relates to attachment and personality style that seem promising for future research aimed at better delineating and informing treatment (Lampe & Malhi, 2018).

AvPD and SP are considered to be closely related conditions, but little is known about the underlying processes related to the social discomfort of subjects with either of the disorders. Because both disorders are associated with interpersonal problems, an attachment perspective was thought to reveal similarities and differences in close relationships between the disorders (Eikenaes, Pedersen, & Wilberg, 2016).

In a study comparing self-reported attachment styles in patients with AvPD and SP, it was expected that patients with AvPD would have more attachment anxiety and would exhibit a fearful attachment style more often compared with individuals with SP. A cross-sectional multisite study was conducted with 90 adult patients with AvPD and SP. Patients with AvPD with and without SP (AvPD group) were compared with patients with SP without AvPD (SP group). Both structured diagnostic interviews and self-reporting questionnaires were used.

The results showed higher levels of attachment anxiety within the AvPD group, especially for the subfactors of anxiety for abandonment and separation frustration. Levels of avoidance did not show a difference between the diagnostic groups. After controlling for symptom disorders and the criteria of other personality disorders, anxiety for abandonment was still associated with AvPD. A fearful attachment style was more frequent among patients with AvPD. The results indicate greater attachment anxiety in AvPD individuals than in people with SP, and the anxiety was most pronounced for the fear of abandonment. This fear of abandonment may play a significant role in the AvPD pathology.

Treatment

Currently, there are no published clinical trials that have examined treatments for co-occurring AvPD and BPD, but for AvPD, cognitive behavioral therapy (CBT) appears to be effective (Salters-Pedneault, 2017). However, avoidant individuals rarely seek treatment because therapy is essentially a setting of "social" interaction, which requires a certain degree of vulnerability to be effective, and vulnerability is what the sufferer tries so hard to avoid.

AvPD is not expected to improve over time without treatment. A major goal in treatment is to establish sufficient rapport between patient and therapist, so that the patient will open up without excessive fear of criticism.

Treatment of AvPD may use various techniques, such as social skills training, cognitive therapy, and exposure therapy, to gradually increase social contacts to where group therapy can be tolerated for practicing social skills (Comer, 2014).

Once people with AvPD are able to overcome the hurdle of embarrassment in entering outside intervention, they may become receptive and benefit from therapy. Several therapeutic approaches, including behavioral, cognitive-behavioral, and psychoanalysis, are successful in treating people with AvPD (Dobbert, 2007).

Some of the particularly promising possibilities in working with individuals with AvPD, as considered by some researchers, include the incorporation of techniques such as video feedback, treatments focused on interpersonal relationships, and intervention strategies associated with traditional CBT (Herbert, 2007).

Some people with a personality disorder may be able to tolerate long-term therapy, but people with the concerns of AvPD typically enter therapy only when they feel overwhelmed by stress, which exacerbates the symptoms of the personality disorder. This shorter-term therapy will usually focus on the immediate difficulties in the person's life. Once the difficulty that brought the person to enter therapy is resolved, the person will leave treatment. Medications may be useful in helping with specific troubling and debilitating symptoms (Bressert, 2017). Some symptoms of AvPD have been found to be reduced through prescription of SSRI antidepressants.

Without treatment, people with AvPD may become resigned to a life of near or total isolation. They may, in turn, develop a second psychiatric disorder, such as substance abuse, or a mood disorder, such as depression.

A published report of a long-time psychodynamic psychotherapy case of a female client with a history of childhood trauma, avoidant attachment style, and AvPD demonstrates how—by applying the concept of "earned security attachment"—the client developed a secure attachment to significant others as her symptoms remitted, and her life improved drastically (Guina, 2016)."Earned security" is defined as "the processes by which individuals overcome malevolent parenting experiences" (Roisman, Padron, Sroufe, & Egeland, 2002, p. 1206).

References

Barends Psychology Practice. (2018). Interesting avoidant personality disorder facts. Retrieved June 6, 2018, from https://www.barendspsychology.com/interesting-avoidant-personality-disorder-facts/

Bayer, L. (2000). *Personality disorders*. Philadelphia, PA: Chelsea House Publishers.

Bressert, S. (2017). Avoidant personality disorder. *Psych Central*. Retrieved December 26, 2017, from https://psychcentral.com /disorders/avoidant-personality-disorder/

Brown, E. J., Heimberg, R. G., & Juster, H. R. (1995). Social phobia subtype and avoidant personality disorder: Effects on severity of social phobia, impairment, and outcome of cognitive behavioral treatment. *Behavior Therapy, 26*(3), 467–486.

Coid, J., Yang, M., Tyrer, P., Roberts, A., & Ullrich, S. (2006). Prevalence and correlates of personality disorder among adults aged 16 to 74 in Great Britain. *British Journal of Psychiatry, 188*, 423–431.

Comer, R. (2014). *Fundamentals of abnormal psychology* (pp. 424–427). New York, NY: Worth Publishers.

Connors, M. E. (1997). The renunciation of love: Dismissive attachment and its treatment. *Psychoanalytic Psychology, 14*, 475–493.

Dobbert, D. L. (2007). *Understanding personality disorders*. Westport, CT: Praeger.

Eikenaes, I., Pedersen, G., & Wilberg, T. (2016). Attachment styles in patients with avoidant personality disorder compared with social phobia. *Psychological Psychotherapy, 89*(3), 245–260. doi:10.1111/papt 12075 Epub 2015 Aug 31.

Fogelson, D., & Nuechterlein, K. (2007). Avoidant personality disorder is a separable schizophrenia-spectrum personality disorder even when controlling for the presence of paranoid and schizotypal personality disorders. *Schizophrenia Research, 91*, 192–199.

Gratz, K. L., & Tull, M. T. (2012). Exploring the relationship between posttraumatic stress disorder and deliberate self-harm: The moderating roles of borderline and avoidant personality disorders. *Psychiatry Research, 199*(1), 19–23.

Guina, J. (2016). The talking cure of avoidant personality disorder remission through earned secure attachment. *American Journal of Psychotherapy, 70*(3), 233–250.

Gunderson, J. G., Shea, M. T., Skodol, A. E., McGlashan, T. H., Morey, L. C., Stout, R. L., ... Keller, M. B. (2000). The collaborative longitudinal personality disorders study: Development, aims, design, and sample characteristics. *Journal of Personality Disorders, 14*(4), 300–315.

Herbert, J. D. (2007). Avoidant personality disorder. In W. O'Donahue, K. A. Fowler, & S. O. Lilienfeld (Eds.), *Personality disorders: Toward the DSM-V* (pp. 279–305). Thousand Oaks, CA: Sage Publications.

Herbert, J. D., Hope, D. A., & Bellack, A. S. (1992). Validity of the distinction between generalized social phobia and avoidant personality disorder. *Journal of Abnormal Psychology, 101*(2), 332–339.

Hoeksema, N. (2014). *Abnormal psychology* (6th ed., p. 275). New York, NY: McGraw Education.

Holt, C. S., Heimberg, B. G., & Hope, D. A. (1992). Avoidant personality disorder and the generalized subtype of social phobia. *Journal of Abnormal Psychology, 101*(2), 318–325.

Kantor, M. (1993, revised 2003). *Distancing: A guide to avoidance and avoidant personality disorder.* Westport, CT: Praeger Publishers.

Kretschmer, E. (1921). *Körperbau und Charakter.* Berlin, Germany: J. Springer.

Lampe, L. I., & Malhi, G. S. (2018). Avoidant personality disorder: Current insights. *Psychology Research & Behavior Management, 11,* 55–66. doi:102147/PR.BM.S12107.3 eCollection 2018

Lenzenweger, M. F., & Clarkin, J. F. (2005). *Major theories of personality disorder.* New York, NY: Guilford Press.

McLean, P. D., & Woody, S. R. (2001). *Anxiety disorders in adults: An evidence-based approach to psychological treatment.* New York, NY: Oxford University Press.

Meyer, B., Ajchenbrenner, M., & Bowles, D. P. (2005). Sensory sensitivity, attachment experiences, and rejection responses among adults with borderline and avoidant features. *Journal of Personality Disorders, 19*(6), 641–658.

Millon, T. (2015). Personality subtypes summary. *Institute for Advanced Studies in Personology and Psychopathology.* Retrieved from http://www.millon.net/taxonomy/summary.htm

Millon, T., & Davis, R. (1996). *Disorders of personality: DSM-IV and beyond* (2nd ed., p. 263). New York, NY: Wiley.

Mulder, R. T., Joyce, P. R., Frampton, C. M., Luty, S. E., & Sullivan, P. F. (2006). Six months of treatment for depression: Outcome and predictors of the course of illness. *The American Journal of Psychiatry, 163,* 95–100.

Nedic, A., Zivanovic, O., & Lisulov, R. (2011). Nosological status of social phobia: Contrasting classical and recent literature. *Current Opinion in Psychiatry, 24*(1), 61–66.

Out of the FOG. (2016). Personality disorders: Avoidant personality disorder (AvPD). Retrieved April 21, 2018, from http://outofthefog.website/personality-disorders-1/2015/12/6/avoidant-personality-disorder-avpd

Reich, J. (2009). Avoidant personality disorder and its relationship to social phobia. *Current Psychiatry Reports, 11*(1), 89–93.

Rettew, D. C. (2008). Avoidant personality disorder. *Emedicine*. Retrieved from http://emedicine.medscape.com

Rettew, D. C., Zanarini, M., Yen, S., Grilo, C., Skodol, A., Shea, T., . . . Gunderson, J. (2003). Childhood antecedents of avoidant personality disorder: A retrospective study. *Journal of the American Academy of Child & Adolescent Psychiatry, 42*(9), 1122–1130. Retrieved August 4, 2010, from http://www.jaacap.com/article /S0890-8567%2809%2961010-8/abstract

Roisman, G. I., Padron, E., Sroufe, L. A., & Egeland, B. (2002). Earned secure attachment status in retrospect and prospect. *Child Development, 73*(4), 1204–1219.

Salters-Pedneault, K. P. (2017). Borderline and avoidant personality disorders: The co-occurrence of BPD and AvPD. *Verywellmind*. Retrieved December 17, 2017, from https://www.verywellmind.com /borderline-and-avoidant-personality-disorder-425419

Schneier, E. R., Spitzer, R. L., Gibbon, M., Feyer, A. J., & Liebowitz, M. R. (1991). The relationship of social phobia subtypes and avoidant personality disorder. *Comprehensive Psychiatry, 32*(6), 496–502.

Sederer, L. I. (2009). *Blueprints psychiatry*. Philadelphia, PA: Wolters Kluwer/Lippincott Williams & Wilkins.

Sutherland, S. M. (2006). Avoidant personality disorder: Causes, frequency, siblings and mortality—morbidity. *Avoidant Personality Disorder*. Armenian Medical Network. Retrieved February 26, 2007, from http://www.health.am/psy/avoidant-personality-disorder-causes/

Tomko, R. L., Trull, T. J., Wood, P. K., & Sher, K. J. (2014). Characteristics of borderline personality disorder in a community sample: Comorbidity, treatment utilization, and general functioning. *Journal of Personality Disorders, 285*, 734–750.

Turner, S. M., Beidel, D. C., Dancu, C. V., & Keys, D. J. (1986). Psychopathology of social phobia and comparison to avoidant personality disorder. *Journal of Abnormal Psychology, 95*(4), 389–394.

Turner, S. M., Beidel, D. C., & Townsley, R. M. (1992). Social phobia: A comparison of specific and generalized subtypes and avoidant personality disorder. *Journal of Abnormal Psychology, 102*(2), 326–331.

Van Velzen, C. J. M. (2002). *Social phobia and personality disorders: Comorbidity and treatment issues*. Groningen: University Library Groningen. (Online version: http://irs.ub.rug.nl/ppn/240921941)

Verheul, R. (2001). Co-morbidity of personality disorders in individuals with substance use disorders. *European Psychiatry, 16*(5), 274–282.

Retrieved from http://www.sciencedirect.com/science/article/pii/S09249 33801005788

Weinbrecht, A., Schulze, L., Boettcher, J., & Renneberg, B. (2016). Avoidant personality disorder: A current review. *Current Psychiatry Reports, 18*(3) 29.

Wood, J. C. (2010). *The cognitive behavioral therapy workbook for personality disorders: A step-by-step program.* Oakland, CA: New Harbinger Publications.

Zimmerman, M., Rothschild, L., & Chelminski, I. (2005). The prevalence of DSM-IV personality disorders in psychiatric outpatients. *The American Journal of Psychiatry, 162*(10), 1911–1918.

CHAPTER 3

Borderline Personality Disorder

Symptoms, Diagnosis, and Incidence

According to the most recent edition of the *Diagnostic and Statistical Manual of Mental Disorders* (*DSM-5*) borderline personality disorder (BPD)—a Cluster B personality disorder—is characterized by a "pervasive pattern of instability of interpersonal relationships, self-image, and affects, and marked impulsivity that begins by early adulthood and is present in a variety of contexts" (p. 663). Individuals with this disorder desperately try to avoid real or imagined abandonment. Their intense abandonment fears lead to inappropriate anger when faced with even time-limited abandonment or unavoidable changes in plans. Impulsive actions, such as self-mutilating or suicidal behavior, may result from trying to avoid the feared abandonment.

Conceptually similar to borderline personality disorder is how the World Health Organization's ICD-10 describes *emotionally unstable personality disorder*, which includes two subtypes: impulsive type and borderline type. Even more subtypes of BPD have been proposed by Theodore Millon (2004), who suggested that individuals diagnosed with BPD may exhibit none, one, or more of the four categories: *discouraged, petulant, impulsive*, and *self-destructive* subtypes.

Arguing that many mental health professionals have difficulty diagnosing BPD on the basis of DSM criteria, which describe a wide variety of behaviors, Marsha Linehan (1993), who developed Dialectical Behavior Therapy, has grouped the symptoms of BPD under five main areas of dysregulation: emotions, behavior, interpersonal relationships, sense of self, and cognition.

Borderline personality disorder has been considered the most important clinical problem on Axis II, and, consequently, most personality disorder research has focused on this category (Paris, 2008). In addition to experiencing extreme mood swings, people with borderline personality disorder may display uncertainty about who they are. As a result, their interests and values can change rapidly.

Emotional dysregulation is considered to be the borderline pattern. A general instability in emotions, interpersonal relationships, cognitive functioning, and in sense of self pervades the individual's character organization. The core emotional trait at the center of the pattern is an *affective lability*, involving unstable and reactive moods, including labile anger and anxiousness, manifested by a lifelong tendency to worry and ruminate. The emotional core often includes hypersensitivity—a tendency to experience everything intensely, with the result that emotions and other forms of stimulation feel intrusive and overwhelming. This emotional core is associated with *cognitive dysregulation*, a tendency toward disorganized or confused thinking. The interpersonal traits of submissiveness and insecure attachment are also part of this pattern. Cognitive disorganization may—in more severe cases—include experiences of depersonalization.

Estimates of the median population prevalence of BPD are 1.6 percent but may be as high as 5.9 percent, according to a 2008 study and the *DSM-5*. In primary care settings, the prevalence of BPD is 6 percent, while it is about 10 percent among outpatient mental health clinic patients and about 20 percent among psychiatric inpatients. BPD appears to be the most prevalent disorder in treatment settings (Bjornlund, 2011).

Borderline personality disorder seems to be more prevalent in females, as 75 percent of diagnoses made are in females. Within older age groups, the prevalence of borderline personality disorder may decrease. Many people are experiencing few of the most extreme symptoms by the time they are in their 40s or 50s.

Timeline

1938   Psychoanalyst Adolf Stern was the first to use the term "borderline."

1959   Melitta Schmideberg, daughter of psychoanalyst Melanie Klein, wrote about the outcome of BPD

1968   Roy Grinker published the first empirical study of borderline patients.

1970   Psychoanalyst Otto Kernberg was the first to use the term "borderline" to describe patients whose symptoms are between psychosis and neurosis. He proposed three levels of character pathology.

1970s   Psychology professor Marsha M. Linehan introduces dialectical behavior therapy, which became a key treatment for borderline personality disorder.

1975   John Gunderson demonstrated that this form of pathology (BPD) could be operationalized with behavioral criteria.

1980   The definition of borderline personality disorder (BPD) was adopted by the *Diagnostic and Statistical Manual of Mental Disorders* (third edition, *DSM-III*).

1994   A ninth criterion for BPD to describe cognitive symptoms was added in the *DSM-IV*.

2007   The National Alliance on Mental Illness adds borderline personality disorder as a research focus.

2009   The U.S. House of Representatives declares May as Borderline Personality Disorder Month, bringing new attention to the disorder.

History

When psychoanalyst Adolf Stern (1938) described borderline personality, he observed that these patients did not progress in therapy; they got worse. This led him to believe that these patients were unsuitable for analytic treatment because their pathology was on a "borderline" between neurosis and psychosis. Their clinical features were seen as "psychic bleeding," inordinate hypersensitivity, and difficulties in reality testing and in relationships.

Melitta Schmideberg wrote about the outcome of treating BPD patients and described their course as "stably unstable"—this was a clinical impression, not a conclusion based on data. The studies of inpatients at the time generally confirmed Schmideberg's description. In a follow-up of 51 patients who had been treated at Chicago's Michael Reese Hospital, Roy Grinker and his group found that after five years, most patients had changed little. Similar findings were reported by Harrison Pope (1983), who studied 33 patients admitted to McLean Hospital in Boston. After five years the patients had not recovered and had not developed additional mental disorders.

In the 1950s, the concept of borderline personality disorder was devised to describe patients who were considered to be on the borderline between neurosis and psychosis. Some researchers thought that borderline personality disorder and schizophrenia were related biologically, with borderline personality disorder being a milder form of schizophrenia (Dolecki, 2012). However, many clinicians disagreed with this "borderline," and the concept evolved into a personality disorder.

Over the next 30 years, there was only sporadic interest in borderline pathology. The three levels of character pathology proposed by Kernberg were a milder (close to "neurosis"), a moderate, and a severe (i.e., borderline) level. However, there were problems with this "borderline personality organization" (BPO) because it was defined on the basis of theories about mental mechanisms rather than on observable behaviors (being entirely psychoanalytical), and the definition of BPO included a very broad group of patients as "borderline." Some clinicians described BPD as "an adjective in search of a noun" (Akiskal, Chen, & Davis, 1985).

This trend was broken when Roy Grinker's study gave more weight to clinical observation than to psychodynamic speculations. Grouping into subcategories was based on observable symptoms (Grinker, Werble, & Dyre, 1968).

A turning point for the acceptance of BPD came with the work of John Gunderson of McLean Hospital and Harvard Medical School. It demonstrated that this disorder could be understood and worked with in the framework of behavioral criteria and that a semistructured interview could yield a reliable diagnosis (Gunderson & Singer, 1975)

Linehan (1993) proposed the theory that BPD develops primarily from *emotional dysregulation* (ED). There is empirical evidence to support the centrality of ED as patients with BPD have more intense emotions to begin with, experience difficulty regulating them, and rapidly shift from one emotion to another (Putnam & Silk, 2005).

Development and Causes

The developmental course of BPD shows considerable variability, with the most common pattern being one of chronic instability in early adulthood, including episodes of serious affective and impulsive dyscontrol and high levels of mental health resource use. The greatest impairment and highest risk of suicide occur in the young-adult years of individuals with the disorder, gradually decreasing with age.

The prognosis for developing BPD is about five times more common among first-degree biological relatives than in the general population. In addition, there is an increased familial risk for substance use disorders, antisocial personality disorder, and depressive or bipolar disorders.

The largest twin study of borderline personality disorder, conducted in 2000, found that 35 percent of individuals with an identical twin diagnosed with BPD share the diagnosis, compared with only 7 percent of fraternal twins, indicating that BPD and other personality disorders are grounded in genetics.

An ongoing twin study in the Netherlands (Trull, 2008) included 711 pairs of siblings and 561 parents who were examined to identify the location of genetic traits that influenced the development of BPD. It was found that genetic material on chromosome 9 was linked to BPD, leading researchers to conclude that a major role in individual differences of BPD features was played by genetic factors. From an earlier study, the same researchers had concluded that 42 percent of variation in BPD features was attributable to genetic factors and 58 percent was due to environmental influences.

It is generally held that the interaction of biological and environmental risk factors reaches a certain critical level of brain dysfunction, which makes the symptoms of BPD observable. This critical disturbance of brain function can be brought about by a large amount of biological risk requiring only a small amount of environmental risk, or low biological risk coupled with high environmental risks, or intermediate levels of both (Friedel, 2010).

Many people with BPD report a history of abuse and neglect, having experienced traumatic life events, or having been exposed to unstable relationships, and there is a strong relationship between child abuse, especially child sexual abuse, and development of BPD. However, causation is still debated.

According to the results of some studies, family breakdown is a risk factor for BPD. But the effects of specific forms of breakdown are not consistent, with some studies reporting an increased incidence and others finding no significant relationship.

Discussion regarding the core features of BPD includes Marsha Linehan's (1993) description of BPD in terms of interpersonal, behavioral, cognitive, and self-dysregulation. She argues that emotional dysregulation is the core feature of borderline pathology, while suggestions from others point to impulsivity as the core feature (Links, Heslegrave, & van Reekum, 1999).

Within the current framework, however, it has been stated that deliberate self-harm and many other impulsive acts are secondary to emotional dysregulation, as suggested earlier. In addition, many of the so-called impulsive acts are actually planned, as some patients apparently anticipate when and how in the future they will harm themselves next. Impulsivity seems to be a more complex concept than is generally recognized (Parker & Bagby, 1997).

Studies have documented typical cases of BPD during adolescence, but it is unknown whether patients with an onset in adolescence have a better or worse course and prognosis than those with later onset. Although it was once thought that "adolescent turmoil" does not present a risk for adult psychopathology, current evidence indicates that it does (Cicchetti & Rogosch, 2002).

Effects and Costs

The most severe risk related to BPD is suicide. It has been estimated that as many as 75 percent of individuals with this affliction will attempt to kill themselves at some point. As many as 10 percent eventually will take their own lives.

Toward the end of the twentieth century, treating sources described borderline patients as repeatedly cutting themselves, trying to hang themselves, or overdosing. Treating staff were often stressed, psychiatrists were frustrated and irritated, and other patients felt both traumatized and neglected due to the hospital units' management problems in handling borderline patients (Dunn & Parry, 1997).

The name "borderline personality disorder" itself has created stigma for those individuals who have been diagnosed with the disorder. Some professionals have been avoiding working with people who have BPD because of the difficulty in diagnosing the complex symptoms.

Patients' behaviors, such as keeping their appointments erratically in spite of repeatedly requiring emergency responses, often aroused negative feelings. These actions were not seen as part of a mental illness but as attention-seeking or acting-out behaviors. In hospitals, BPD patients were regarded as "help-rejecting complainers," and at best, a diagnosis of BPD was a statement of therapeutic pessimism.

At times, BPD has been mistaken for bipolar mood disorder, both in name and symptoms. Some of the confusion is due to the similarity of symptoms and because there is more information and public attention focused on bipolar mood disorder. However, the mood swings for BPD are more consistent than those for bipolar mood disorder, which tend to occur in cycles or as the result of certain situations that have recently occurred. With BPD, on the other hand, mood swings occur as part of the person's general pattern of behaviors rather than as result of situations and cycles (Dolecki, 2012).

People afflicted with borderline personality disorder typically use a high amount of health care resources; BPD is estimated to account for 20 percent of psychiatric hospitalizations.

In Society

Since the 1960s, the credibility of individuals with PD has been questioned, based on two main issues, dissociation episodes and lying, which are both commonly believed to constitute key components of the disorder. A 1999 study reported decreased specificity of autobiographical memory in patients with BPD. Furthermore, the belief that lying is a distinguishing characteristic of BPD can make a difference in the quality of care that people with this diagnosis receive in the legal and health care systems. Even within the mental health community, BPD can be a stigmatizing diagnosis. Another defining characteristic of BPD— manipulative behavior to obtain nurturance—has been assumed to be intentional behavior. Thus, characteristics connected with the diagnosis of BPD may contribute to stigmatizing the people living with the diagnosis. Additionally, dramatic portrayals of people with BPD in movies and other forms of social media contribute to the stigma in the public eye surrounding BPD.

Comparing traditional and modern societies, some researchers may conclude that the conditions in traditional societies are not conducive to the development of BPD because people who are unusually emotional and impulsive will be contained by powerful social structures. However, growing up in modern society can contain risk factors for encouraging BPD. Everything in modern society encourages young individuals to separate from parents and assigns importance to peer groups. If one's peers are experimenting with drugs or sex, one is likely to succumb to that influence. Young individuals who are emotional and impulsive may be trapped in a path that runs out of control. These characteristics give BPD the foundation of a *socially sensitive* disorder, one whose prevalence changes with time and circumstances (Paris, 2008).

Up Close

Thirty-six-year-old Rachel became a patient at a mental health clinic after ingesting a large amount of various pills in a serious suicide attempt.

Rachel had difficulty getting along with her mother, who never approved of her. After a secret marriage at a young age, Rachel's new husband died in a traffic accident, and Rachel's pregnancy ended in a miscarriage. Obtaining employment in a veterinarian's office, she returned to her hometown without telling her parents about her marriage and pregnancy. She never entered into another romantic relationship with a man but engaged in friendships with women, some of them being intense. Although brief, Rachel's intense mood swings led to breakups with several of her female friends. Being hypersensitive to any type of criticism, she invited it by complaining how incompetent she was in so many areas of her life. She never stopped blaming herself for losing the baby after her husband's death. To her, this was evidence that she was not strong enough to lead a normal woman's life. But her depressed moods were interrupted with livelier and almost giddy mood states when she spent time with some of her female friends. At other times, she had some angry outbursts at work, never toward any of the animals—rather, the animals' owners became the target of her fury. She blamed the owners for many of the animals' illnesses that brought them to the clinic. After a while Rachel turned to alcohol to deal with her mood swings at home. Her friends distanced themselves from Rachel because of her argumentativeness.

Unfortunately, the alcohol use also loosened her inhibitions about expressing anger at work. Her outbursts became more frequent until her employer fired her. This was the point when she turned to suicide. She had been evicted from her apartment due to her quarrelsome attitudes toward her neighbors, who had united against her and convinced the landlord to force her to move. With no job and no home, she was forced to return to her now-widowed mother's house. Rachel's mother agreed to let her live with her in exchange for taking care of the house and the mother's needs. In addition, Rachel's mother insisted that Rachel get rid of her beloved cat.

Initially, following her suicide attempt, Rachel had been diagnosed with bipolar disorder. However, tests and her history made a diagnosis of BPD more reasonable.

At Work

Individuals diagnosed with BPD often experience intense emotions, making it difficult for them to control their focus and concentration. In work situations these difficulties may lead to impaired job performance.

In general, BPD has been related to lower functioning and disability, even when socioeconomic status, medical conditions, and psychiatric problems were controlled. Furthermore, it is more common for females with BPD to experience disabilities than for men with BPD.

The black-and-white thinking of people with BPD seems to find reinforcement in certain professional fields. Some of these fields might be in human industries, such as social work and clinical therapy, while others might be in criminal justice fields, such as police officers, military officers, or prison guards. Generally, these fields entail positions and situations for power and control over others, being in the "good guy" role, caring for others, or putting bad guys in their place (Dolecki, 2012).

However, people with BPD often experience difficulty focusing on what they are supposed to be doing and may not get their work duties done on time, leaving coworkers to pick up the slack, which leads to resentment among the coworkers.

Up Close

Jane, a 29-year-old nurse, had been having problems with emotional outbursts since adolescence, but she was able to remain employed in her profession mainly by working night shifts. She had a few brief hospitalizations for suicide threats but always returned to her job and never made a real suicide attempt. In nursing school, Jane had been one of the best students. During that time, she was involved in many brief romantic relationships. Some of her partners were addicted to drugs, and some even had criminal records. Their lifestyle, though quite different from that of a nurse, was exciting to her and seemed to fit with her own emotional instability.

Unfortunately, over the years her emotional outbursts began to occur at work as well as in her personal life. There were angry outbursts with her colleagues, and on several occasions, she stormed off the ward in the middle of the night. She lost her job at the hospital, and her reputation spread to other care centers. For a while she worked as a home care nurse, taking care of private patients in their homes. Her anger flared up again, and she finally had to be removed from a patient's home by the police, who were called by a family member of her patient.

Jane was lucky that the family did not press charges, but her nursing career was over, and she applied for disability.

In Relationships

Individuals with BPD experience *affective instability*, which means that their moods can change by the day or by the hour, and shifts from depression to anger are particularly common, putting a lot of stress on any relationship.

People with BPD can be very sensitive to the way they are treated by others. It ranges from feeling gratitude and intense joy at perceived expressions of kindness to anger or intense sadness at perceived criticism or hurtfulness. Their feelings about others can shift rapidly from love or admiration to anger or dislike when disappointed or threatened with loss of esteem in the eyes of someone they value or the threat of losing someone. This shift from idealizing others to devaluating them is sometimes called splitting. Splitting, combined with intense mood disturbances can undermine relationships with family, friends, and coworkers. Equally rapid changes can occur in the person's self-image.

Although they may strongly desire intimacy with others, people with BPD tend to demonstrate insecure, avoidant, or ambivalent behaviors or fearfully preoccupied attachment patterns in relationships. Quite often, the world is viewed as dangerous and malevolent. Romantic relationships are characterized by conflict and increased levels of chronic stress, as well as by decreased satisfaction on the part of romantic partners. In addition, people with BPD often have difficulty understanding their own identity, such as not exactly knowing what they value, prefer, believe, and enjoy. And they are often unsure about their long-term goals for relationships and jobs, leading to feeling "empty" and "lost."

It has been pointed out that in many ways, the traits and temperaments linked to BPD run contrary to gender stereotypes about how men should be. This may create shame in men with BPD. In order to save face, these men may deny their insecurity and sensitivity and be willing to accept a label of "antisocial personality," "impulse control disorder," or "depression" because these disorders sound more manly than borderline personality disorder. These "preferred" diagnoses can provide a convenient "cover" for the real issues, and some clinicians have resorted to use MBPD as a diagnostic unit for men afflicted with BPD (Nowinski, 2014).

Spouses of BPD patients often see themselves as walking on eggshells, trying to please their partners and avoid arguments. "Being married to someone with BPD is heaven one minute, hell the next," according to the spouse of a BPD patient (Mason & Kreger, 2010, p. 11).

Up Close

At age 32, Leonard was confronted by police as they attempted to remove him from his home. Over the police officer's voice, he could hear Susan sob and yell, "Take him out, please take him out of here!" This was the second time the police had responded to a 911 call at this location within the past 10 months. Today's call had been in response to Leonard's violent outburst, which ended with him throwing a chair across the living room, striking the wall next to the door. Susan told the officer Leonard had aimed the chair at her when she was trying to leave the room.

Susan and Leonard shared *a four-year turbulent relationship. It had been immediate mutual attraction when they met at a friend's wedding. Their dating history started on the day of the friend's wedding, and six months later they held their own wedding. Leonard worked in an accounting firm but did not seem very self-assured. However, he liked it when Susan tried to build up his self-esteem by repeatedly telling him that he was doing very well.*

Apparently, Leonard had expected that Susan would spend all her free time with him, but Susan did not want to give up seeing her friends from time to time. Leonard did not hide his disappointment, and sometimes, upon her return home from an evening with her friends, he tried to put a guilt trip on her, pointing out her negligence in considering the significance of marriage. On one of those evenings, Susan decided to spend the night in their little guest room instead of their bedroom. Leonard was shocked. Several times during the night he got up and walked around their apartment, mumbling and sighing. The next morning, Leonard told Susan that he had not been able to sleep without her and that he felt abandoned by her. Susan tried to reassure him that she loved him, and she moved her nightgown back into the bedroom before she left for work.

For a while, things were calm, until Susan decided to meet her friends again right after work. By the time she came home, Leonard was pacing the floor, accusing her of avoiding his phone calls. It turned out that Susan had put her cell phone on silent when she was with her friends, and Leonard's calls went to her voice mail. This time Leonard's emotions turned to anger. When Susan tried to evade his accusations by going to the bathroom, Leonard grabbed her arms and stopped her from moving away, letting his angry voice filled with complaints and accusations rain down on her. She finally managed to get free from his grip and went into the bathroom, locking the door behind her. After her shower she went straight into the guest room and locked that door. Leonard banged on the door for a while, yelling angrily, but finally gave up and went to bed. He apologized the next morning. Leonard's behavior became more unstable, begging for love one moment but then, when his requests did not bring immediate relief, turning to depression, anger, and then to violent outbursts until the time when Susan called 911.

Theory and Research

Among the stronger symptoms of borderline personality disorder is a high sensitivity to rejection. The brain's executive function seems to be the mediating agent in the relationship between rejection sensitivity and

BPD symptoms. A group of cognitive processes, such as planning, working memory, attention, and problem solving might be the mechanism through which BPD symptoms are impacted by rejection sensitivity. As demonstrated in a 2008 study, the relationship between an individual's rejection sensitivity and BPD symptoms was stronger when executive function was lower, and, conversely, the relationship was weaker with higher executive function. This would suggest that high executive function might help protect individuals with high rejection sensitivity against the symptoms of BPD. Such findings could be useful when expressed to the patient during treatment as a possibility for reducing the impact of the disorder on the individual's discomfort to some degree.

Findings of another study in 2012 implied that greater impulsivity in people with BPD might be linked to problems in their working memory.

Two types of parental behavior—neglectful and overprotective—have been associated with borderline personality disorder. Those studies were based on retrospective recall of childhood events and, as such, may have been biased by the effect of psychopathology. However, a community study, which used more objective information about abuse and neglect (court records), reported similar findings. In other studies 25–73 percent of patients with borderline personality disorder reported severe physical abuse.

The relationship between sexual abuse and borderline personality disorder has perhaps received the most attention. Upward of 70 percent of patients reported a history of that type of abuse. These findings led to the conclusion that trauma is a major etiological factor for borderline personality disorder. Other evidence, however, does not support such a conclusion. A meta-analysis of 21 studies involving 2,479 individuals revealed only a moderate association between childhood sexual abuse and borderline personality disorder. The conclusion of the literature reviews suggested that about one-third of patients with borderline personality disorder reported severe abuse involving an incestuous perpetrator, severe sexual abuse, and high frequency or long duration.

It has been pointed out that empirical research revealing the broad array of features delineating BPD meet the criteria for other personality disorders as well. This convergence has been used to suggest that the *DSM-IV*'s BPD is an artificially circumscribed category to distinguish it from other diagnoses. Therefore, it appears that the disorder may be more an indication of severe personality dysfunction than a distinct diagnostic entity (Berkelowitz & Tarnopolsky, 1993).

Although most personality disorder research has focused on this category, some criticism has been expressed, stating that as long as categories of mental disorder are based on clinical observation instead of on biological markers, such as blood tests or imaging findings, validity will remain weak (Paris, 2008).

John Gunderson at McLean Hospital developed the Diagnostic Interview for Borderline Patients (DIB), which was later revised by Mary Zanarini (DIB-R) (Zanarini et al., 1989). It is a semistructured interview assessing people's conditions in the four domains of BPD pathology (affective, cognitive, impulsive, and interpersonal). Each domain is scored separately with a maximum score of 10, and 8/10 being the cutoff for BPD.

Trait psychologists prefer *dimensional* models—constructs that describe continuous variations over sharp categories—and within their approach, BPD can be described through personality trait profiles rather than as categories. Their most widely used measure is the five-factor model of personality (FFM) (Costa & Widiger, 2001) which describes personality on five broad dimensions: neuroticism, extraversion, openness to experience, agreeableness, and conscientiousness. People with BPD and other personality disorders tend to have high scores on neuroticism and low scores on agreeableness and conscientiousness.

The fact that most personality disorders tend to be continuous with normal personality traits is one of the main arguments in support of a dimensional system, as research in community and clinical populations usually doesn't show any sharp separation between pathological and normal personality traits (Livesley, Jang, & Vernon, 1998). The principle of continuity between traits and disorders is relevant to most of the Axis II categories.

While dimensions are good for describing the traits that underlie BPD, they cannot account for its symptoms, and the disorder cannot be understood without understanding its trait domains (Paris, 2008).

Studies of comorbidity have shown that at some point in their lives, 75 percent of people with BPD meet criteria for mood disorders, especially major depression and bipolar I. Nearly 75 percent meet criteria for an anxiety disorder, nearly 73 percent for substance abuse or dependency, and about 40 percent for PTSD. It is noteworthy that less than half of patients with BPD experience PTSD during their lives because it challenges the theory that BPD and PTSD are the same disorder.

The types of comorbid conditions in people with BPD show marked gender differences—a higher percentage of females with BPD meet criteria for PTSD and eating disorders, while criteria for substance-use disorders are met by a higher percentage of males. Criteria for a diagnosis of ADHD were met by 38 percent of participants with BPD in one study, and in another study, 6 of 41 participants (15%) met the criteria for an autism spectrum disorder.

At some point in their lives, more than two-thirds of people diagnosed with BPD also meet the criteria for another Axis II personality disorder. For instance, in a 2008 study, the rate was 73.9 percent. The most common comorbid Axis II disorders, with a prevalence of 50.4 percent in people with BPD, were Cluster A disorders, such as paranoid, schizoid, and schizotypal personality disorder.

Comorbidity rates with other Cluster B personality disorders have an overall prevalence of 49.2 percent in people with BPD, with narcissistic being 38.9 percent, antisocial 13.7 percent, and histrionic 10.3 percent.

Research asking study participants to identify various emotional states from observing human faces and their expressions found that some BPD patients are unusually sensitive to facial expressions and are particularly accurate in identifying negative emotions (Frank & Hoffman, 1986), while other BPD patients were hypersensitive to faces expressing fear (Wagner & Linehan, 1999), whereas still other BPD patients experienced neutral faces as threatening; with the use of functional magnetic resonance imaging, the research found that the responses were associated with increased reactivity in the amygdala (Donegan et al., 2003).

In a special study of men recruited through advertisements in an alternative newspaper, it was found that in most respects, men with BPD were identical to women with the disorder; the only difference was that, unlike females, 10 percent of the male sample was actively homosexual.

A study focusing on people aged 18 to 35 who committed suicide revealed that one-third of this cohort suffered from BPD, and many of the suicides were men who were not in treatment. A correlation between separation or loss early in life and suicide completion was observed. However, in a larger study involving 120 patients with BPD, 70 patients who committed suicide did not confirm the finding of early loss as a factor; instead, substance abuse seemed to be a predictor of completion.

Some studies have linked the development of personality disorders with brain abnormalities, which can be identified by brain imaging techniques. For instance, amygdala hyperactivity had been observed in some cases of borderline personality disorder (Donegan et al., 2003).

It has been observed that in people with borderline personality disorder, the hippocampus is smaller, as it is in people with posttraumatic stress disorder (PTSD), but unlike PTSD, in BPD the amygdala also tends to be smaller. One study found unusually strong activity in the left amygdalas of people with BPD when they experienced and saw displays of negative emotions. As the amygdala generates all emotions—pleasant and unpleasant—this strong activity could explain the unusual strength and longevity of sadness, fear, anger, and shame people with BPD experience and sense in others.

However, contrary to results of earlier studies, individuals with BPD in another study were observed to show less activation in the amygdala with increased negative emotionality than the control group, leading to the explanation that people with BPD seem to be "set up" by their brains to have strong emotional experiences in their lives.

Other brain abnormalities observed in people with BPD include less activity in the prefrontal cortex upon recalling memories of abandonment and elevated cortisol production, indicating a hyperactive hypothalamic-pituitary-adrenal axis (HPA axis), causing people with BPD a greater biological stress response, possibly explaining their greater vulnerability to irritability. An increased cortisol production is also associated with a greater risk of suicidal behavior.

A 2008 study comparing the brain function of BPD and non-BPD individuals playing a competitive game showed lesser activity in the BPD players' anterior insula, the part of the brain that is involved in emotional responses to all kinds of situations. Scientists speculate that this demonstrates why people with BPD have problems with trust.

Another study, in 2009, used magnetic resonance imaging to demonstrate that parts of the brain that were active in healthy people when responding to disturbing emotional scenes were inactive in those with BPD. This would indicate that people with BPD are not able to use those parts of the brain to help regulate their emotions (like healthy people do), and it may explain why their emotional responses are so extreme.

Research published in 2013 has highlighted two patterns of brain activity that may be causing the emotional dysregulation found in BPD. There seems to be an increased activity in the brain circuits that, when it is coupled with reduced activation of the brain circuits that normally regulate these painful emotions, brings about an operative dysfunction in the frontolimbic regions and is thus responsible for the experience of heightened emotional discomfort. However, the specific regions vary from individual to individual, requiring further analysis of more neuroimaging studies.

Thought suppression, or conscious attempts to avoid thinking certain thoughts, was found in a 2005 study to mediate the relationship between emotional vulnerability and BPD symptoms, but a later study indicated that the relationship between emotional vulnerability and BPD symptoms is not necessarily mediated by thought processes. Instead, this study found that thought suppression influences the relationship between an invalidating environment and BPD symptoms.

Other research suggests that opioids may play a role in some personality disorders. For instance, a 2009 study found that people with BPD had more receptors for opioids in the brain but lower levels of the chemicals themselves. Experts have speculated that the self-harm tendencies of BPD patients may be a result of this imbalance.

Based on studies that have shown that people with BPD have an increased capacity to read people's facial expressions, researchers believe that increased levels of oxytocin, a hormone stimulated by the pituitary gland, may contribute to their heightened reaction to other people's moods or emotions. This ability to read the emotions of others may be an asset in some work situations.

Many studies report that almost 25 percent of people diagnosed with BPD are women; mental health professionals use this diagnosis more frequently with women than with men, even when both sexes have the same symptoms.

A 2010 brain imaging study confirmed research suggesting that people with BPD process pain stimuli differently than people without personality disorders, giving new insight into the reasons behind cutting and other self-harm behaviors common among BPD patients.

According to some theorists, one of the defense mechanisms employed by borderline individuals is *splitting*. BPD persons learn to separate their "good" selves from their "bad" selves, with the effect that the distance between these two sources of identity becomes increasingly larger. The "part objects" (good and bad) are psychological substitutes for the whole person, who has both strengths and flaws. The idealized self exists in stark contrast to the villainous bad self, who seems to have no redeeming qualities. This delusional way of seeing oneself and the world develops into a habit used to defend the person with BPD from rejection and disappointment. In reality, however, this defense sets up the borderline person for repeated disillusionment. As new people enter their lives, the individuals with BPD first worship them as being perfect, but then, with time, when they prove to have flaws, they devalue and reject them. At the same time, individuals with BPD are not aware that their own selves are split and that they cannot recognize significant portions of their personality. And this makes self-improvement impossible (Bayer, 2000).

In a 2008 study of patients hospitalized for deliberate self-harm, 64 percent of those aged 45 to 74 and 58.5 percent of those aged 15 to 24 were found to have a personality disorder. The most common type of personality disorder found in the younger group (28.6%) was BPD. As mentioned earlier, an estimated 65 to 75 percent of people with BPD attempt suicide; roughly 10 percent succeed (Bjornlund, 2011).

Treatment

BPD is the most common personality disorder among people in treatment; 30 to 60 percent of patients with personality disorders have a diagnosis of BPD. However, there has been a history of resistance by clinicians to making a diagnosis of BPD. This opposition may, in part, reflect difficulties in treatment. As has been reasoned, BPD is highly comorbid with other disorders, especially depression, and therefore, the comorbidity should be treated rather than PBD (Paris, 2008).

About half of all BPD patients experience hallucinations (mostly auditory) as well as other cognitive symptoms, such as subdelusional paranoid feelings. These clinically important characteristics require specific management (Yee, Korner, McSwiggan, Meares, & Stevenson 2005).

Currently, the treatment of choice for BPD is long-term psychotherapy, in particular, dialectical behavior therapy and psychodynamic approaches; however, the effects are small. Randomized controlled trials have shown that dialectical behavioral therapy (DBT), developed by Marsha Linehan specifically to treat BPD, may be an effective treatment modality. DBT and mentalization-based therapy (MBT), which share many similarities, seem to be the most effective. DBT combines aspects from several other treatment approaches with the key element of helping patients accept themselves as they are. DBT integrates traditional cognitive behavioral therapy (CBT) elements with mindfulness, acceptance, and techniques to increase a person's stress tolerance and emotional control. According to some research, mindfulness meditation may bring about favorable structural changes in brain structures that are associated with BPD. In addition, improvement in BPD-characteristic symptoms seems to have resulted from mindfulness-based interventions.

Early outcome research of BPD at Chicago's Michael Reese Hospital and at McLean Hospital in Boston showed that five-year follow-up assessments did not reflect any changes in the patients' conditions.

The Chestnut Lodge study monitored a large number of patients, establishing a reliable baseline diagnosis. Of the patients treated between 1950 and 1975 at Chestnut Lodge, a small private psychiatric hospital in Rockville, MD, specializing in long-term residential treatment, 72 percent were followed up an average of 15 years after the beginning of their therapy. Most patients had improved significantly, with the mean global assessment of functioning (GAF) score of 64, representing mild impairment. It was observed that the BPD patients functioned best in the second decade after discharge. Only 3 percent of the patients had committed suicide (McGlasha, 1984; 1986).

In summary, although using different samples and methodology, four studies published in the 1980s with the 15-year outcome of BPD patients obtained almost identical results. Concerning the long-term risk of completed suicide, the 15-year studies showed greater improvement than the earlier 5-year studies.

A 27-year follow-up study revealed a 10.3 percent rate of completed suicide, with almost twice as many female patients as male patients involved. The mean age at suicide was 37.3 years, which indicates that suicide completions occur late in the course of the illness, even though attempts at suicide commonly occur in patients in their 20s.

A randomized comparison of group therapy and individual psychotherapy for BPD patients, consisting of 25 sessions of weekly therapy, followed by five biweekly sessions, showed that both conditions led to significant improvement. During the first five sessions, approximately 30 percent of patients terminated group treatment. Although this rate is lower than normally reported for treatments of personality disorder, it is higher than usual for group therapy (Munroe-Blum & Marziali, 1995).

Medications used for personality disorders include antidepressants for treating impulsivity and anticonvulsant drugs used for borderline or histrionic patients to help them balance intense emotions and reduce impulsive outbursts.

According to a 2010 review by the Cochrane collaboration, no medications demonstrate promise for the core symptoms of BPD, such as chronic feelings of emptiness, identity disturbance, and abandonment, although some medications may impact isolated symptoms associated with BPD or some of the symptoms of comorbid conditions. A more recent (2017) review, examining the evidence published since the 2010 review, stated that the evidence of effectiveness of medication for BPD remains mixed and highly compromised by suboptimal study design.

Of the typical antipsychotic medications studied in connection with BPD, haloperidol was found to possibly reduce anger, and flupenthixol may reduce the likelihood of suicidal behavior. One trial found that among the atypical antipsychotics, aripiprazole may be effective in reducing interpersonal problems and impulsivity.

A 2009 review of BPD individuals' treatment history revealed that 34 percent of those patients were initially misdiagnosed, and other data indicate an average lapse of five years between the time when a person reaches out for medical help and the time when BPD is accurately diagnosed.

A longitudinal study tracking the symptoms of people diagnosed with BPD showed that 34.5 percent achieved remission within two years from the beginning of the study. Within four years, remission was achieved by 49.4 percent of the participants, and 68.6 percent had achieved remission within six years. By the end of the study, 73.5 percent of the participants were in remission. Furthermore, of those who recovered from symptoms, only 5.9 percent experienced recurrences. Ten years from baseline, in a later study (during a hospitalization of the subjects), 86 percent of patients were sustained in a stable recovery from symptoms. But a 2005 study shows that 88 percent of BPD patients no longer met the criteria for the disorder 10 years after they started treatment.

References

Akiskal, H. S., Chen, S. E., & Davis, G. C. (1985). Borderline: An adjective in search of a noun. *Journal of Clinical Psychiatry, 46,* 41–48.

Bayer, L. (2000). *Personality disorders.* Philadelphia, PA: Chelsea House Publishers.

Berkelowitz, M., & Tarnopolsky, A. (1993). The validity of borderline personality disorder: An updated review of recent research. In P. Tyrer & G. Stein (Eds.), *Personality disorder reviewed* (pp. 90–112). London: Gaskell.

Bjornlund, L. (2011). *Personality disorders.* San Diego, CA: Reference Point Press.

Chapman, A. L., & Gratz, K. L. (2007). *The borderline personality disorder survival guide: Everything you need to know about living with BPD.* Oakland, CA: New Harbinger Publications.

Cicchetti, D., & Rogosch, F. A. (2002). A developmental psychopathology perspective on adolescence. *Journal of Consulting and Clinical Psychology, 70,* 6–20.

Costa, P. T., Jr., & Widiger, T. A. (2001). Using the five-factor model to represent the DSM-IV personality disorders: An expert consensus approach. *Journal of Abnormal Psychology, 11*(3), 401–412.

Dolecki, C. M. (2012). *The everything guide to borderline personality disorder.* Avon, MA: Adams Media.

Donegan, N. H., Sanislow, C. A., Blumberg, H. P., Fulbright, R. K., Lacadie, C., Skudlarski, P., . . . Wexler, B. F. (2003). Amygdala hyperactivity in borderline personality disorder: Implications for emotional dysregulation, *Biological Psychiatry, 54,* 1284–1293.

Dunn, M., & Parry, G. (1997). A reformulated care plan approach to caring for people with Borderline Personality Disorder in a community mental health service setting. *Clinical Psychology Forum, 104,* 19–22.

Frank, H., & Hoffman, N. (1986). Borderline empathy: An empirical investigation. *Comprehensive Psychiatry, 27,* 387–395.

Grinker, R. R., Werble, B., & Dyre, R. C. (1968). *The borderline patient.* New York, NY: Basic Books.

Linehan, M. N. (1993). *Cognitive-behavioral treatment of borderline personality disorder.* New York, NY: Guilford Press.

Links, P. S., Heslegrave, R., & van Reekum, R. (1999). Impulsivity: Core aspect of borderline personality disorder. *Journal of Personality Disorders, 13,* 1–9.

Livesley, W. J., Jang, K. L., & Vernon, P. A. (1998). Phenotypic and genetic structure of traits delineating personality disorder. *Archives of General Psychiatry, 55,* 941–948.

Mason, P. T., & Kreger, R. (2010). *Stop walking on eggshells: Taking your life back. When someone you care about has borderline personality disorder.* Oakland, CA: New Harbinger.

McGlashan, T. H. (1984). The Chestnut Lodge follow-up study I. Follow-up methodology and study sample. *Archives of General Psychiatry, 41(6)* 573–585.

McGlashan, T. H. (1986). The Chestnut Lodge follow-up study III. Long-term outcomes of Borderline Personalities. *Archives of General Psychiatry, 43(1),* 20–30.

Millon, T. (2004). *Personality disorders in modern life.* Hoboken, NJ: John Wiley and Sons.

Munroe-Blum, H., & Marziali, E. (1995). A controlled trial of short-term group treatment for borderline personality disorder. *Journal of Personality Disorders, 9,* 190–198.

Nowinski, J. (2014). *Hard to love: Understanding and overcoming male borderline personality disorder.* Las Vegas, NV: Central Recovery Press.

Paris, Joel. (2008). *Treatment of borderline personality disorder: A guide to evidence-based practice.* New York, NY: The Guilford Press.

Parker, J. D. A., & Bagby, R. M. (1997). Impulsivity in adults: A critical review of measurement approaches. In C. D. Webster & M. A. Jackson (Eds.), *Impulsivity: Theory, assessment, and treatment* (pp. 142–157). New York, NY: Guilford Press.

Pope, H. G., Jonas, J. M., & Hudson, J. I. (1983). The validity of DSM-III borderline personality disorder. *Archives of General Psychiatry, 40,* 23–30.

Putnam, E., & Silk, K. (2005). Emotional dysregulation and the development of borderline personality disorder. *Development and Psychopathology, 17,* 899–925.

Schmideberg, M. (1959). The borderline patient. In S. Arieti (Ed.), *The American handbook of psychiatry* (Vol. 1, pp. 398–416). New York, NY: Basic Books.

Startup, M., Jones, B., Heard, H., Swales, M., Williams, J. M. G., & Jones, R. S. P. (1999). Autobiographical memory and dissociation in borderline personality disorder. *Psychological Medicine, 29*(6), 1397–1404.

Stern, A. (1938). Psychoanalytic investigation of and therapy in the borderline group of neuroses, *Psychoanalytic Quarterly, 7,* 467–489.

Trull, T. (2008). Possible genetic causes of borderline personality disorder identified. University of Missouri-Columbia. *Science News* Dec. 20, 2018, Sciencedaily.com

Wagner, A. W., & Linehan, M. M. (1999). Facial expression recognition ability among women with borderline personality disorder: Implications for emotion regulation? *Journal of Personality Disorders, 13,* 329–344.

Yee, L., Korner, J., McSwiggan, S., Meares, R. A., & Stevenson, J. (2005). Persistent hallucinations in borderline personality disorders. *Comprehensive Psychiatry, 46,* 147–382.

Zanarini, M. C., Gunderson, J. G., Frankenburg, F. R., & Chauncey, D. L. (1989). The revised Diagnostic Interview for Borderlines: Discriminating BPD from other Axis II disorders. *Journal of Personality Disorders, 3*(1), 10–18.

CHAPTER 4

Dependent Personality Disorder

Symptoms, Diagnosis, and Incidence

A pervasive and excessive need to be taken care of, combined with clinging behavior and fears of separation, which starts in early adulthood, is the basic or essential feature of dependent personality disorder (DPD), formerly known as *asthenic personality disorder*. The submissive and dependent behaviors are attempts to elicit caregiving and are based on the person's self-perception of not being able to function adequately without the help of others.

Having great difficulty making everyday decisions without excessive advice and reassurance, people with DPD tend to be passive, allowing other people to take the initiative and assume responsibility for most areas of their lives. This need for assistance from others goes beyond age-appropriate and situation-appropriate requests for help.

Fear of losing support or approval keeps individuals with DPD from expressing disagreement with others, especially those they are dependent on. Rather than risk losing the support of people they are dependent on, individuals with this disorder will agree with issues even if they feel the issues are wrong. Because of their lack of self-confidence, they have difficulty initiating projects or doing things independently. Usually they will wait for others to start a project, believing that others will be better able to do it. Due to their dependence on others to handle their affairs, people with this disorder will not learn the skills necessary for independent functioning, and thus they will perpetuate the path of dependency. In their intent to ensure assistance, individuals with DPD may go to excessive lengths, to the point of volunteering for unpleasant tasks, if they believe this will secure the needed support.

The end of a close relationship may lead those with the disorder to urgently seek another relationship to continue to provide the care and support they need, thus at times becoming quickly and indiscriminately attached to another caregiving individual. Dependent people suffer from low self-esteem and may belittle their own abilities. Consequently, pessimism and self-doubt are common among these individuals.

Firm evidence about the percentage of men and women who suffer from this disorder is generally lacking, although in mental health clinics, it is one of the most commonly encountered personality disorders, occurring at approximately the same rate in men and in women.

Prevalence estimates of DPD based on a probability subsample from Part II of the National Comorbidity Survey Replication were 0.6 percent, while data from the 2001–2002 National Epidemiologic Survey on Alcohol and Related Conditions (NESARC) yielded prevalence estimates of 0.49 percent. Another estimate suggests that approximately 1 percent of the general adult population suffers from DPD, with women developing the problem more frequently than men (Torgersen, Kringlen, & Cramer, 2001). One source reported a 0.6 percent occurrence of DPD in women as compared to 0.4 percent in men (Beitz, 2006). Other studies report similar occurrence rates among males and females, but in clinical settings, this disorder has been diagnosed more frequently in females than in males. However, according to some research, this is largely due to behavioral differences in interviews and self-reporting rather than an actual difference in prevalence between the sexes (Bornstein, 1996).

Timeline

1913 Emil Kraepelin characterized the dependent individual as "shiftless" in his book *Psychiatrie: Ein Lehrbuch* (Psychiatry: A Textbook).

1923 K. Schneider referred to dependent persons as "weak-willed" in *Die psychopathischen Persönlichkeiten* (The Psychopathic Personalities). This negative view was propagated by early psychoanalytic theorists.

1927 K. Abraham wrote "The Influence of Oral Criticism on Character Formation."

1945   O. Fenichel wrote *The Psychoanalytic Neurosis* (New York, NY: W. W. Norton).

1945   Karen Horney described dependent persons as having a pervasive feeling of their own weakness and helplessness, their self-esteem rising and falling with the approval and disapproval of others.

1947   Erich Fromm provided a more articulate description of the dependent personality.

1947   Harry Stack Sullivan described dependent persons as obedient children of dominating parents.

History

The former name of this disorder was asthenic personality disorder, from the Greek word *astheneia*, meaning weak, indicating a lack or loss of strength.

Within classical psychoanalytic theory, the conceptualization of dependency is directly related to Freud's oral psychosexual stage of development. It was thought that frustration or overgratification resulted in an oral fixation and in an oral type of character, marked by feeling dependent on others for nurturance and by behaviors representative of the oral stage. The focus on a drive-based approach of dependency was changed in later psychoanalytic theories to the recognition of the importance of early relationships and establishing separation from the early caregivers. As the exchanges between the caregiver and the child become internalized, the nature of these interactions becomes part of the concepts of the self and others.

Many researchers—Kraepelin in 1913, Schneider in 1923, Abraham in 1927, Fenichel in 1945, and others—had discussed at length the clinical implications of exaggerated dependency needs. Later theoreticians and clinical researchers suggested that dependency may be a risk factor for certain psychological disorders, hypothesizing links between dependency and depression. But the concept of the dependent personality was given only passing mention in the *DSM-I*. Actually, the *DSM-I* precursor of DPD was a subtype of the passive-aggressive personality, identified as "passive-aggressive personality, passive-dependent type." Strangely enough, the concept of the dependent personality received even less attention in the *DSM-II*. Finally, researchers conceptualized exaggerated dependency needs as a form of psychopathology in and of itself. It was not until the

DSM-III and the *DSM-IIIR* that a full-fledged diagnostic category of DPD was included. The nine symptoms required for a diagnosis of DPD fall into two broad areas: behavioral and affective (Bornstein, 1993).

In the 1950s, some researchers suggested that exaggerated or unexpressed dependency needs would result in the individual's risk for physical illness. Alexander's (1950) work on the psychodynamics of psychosomatic disorders indicated that when the expression of dependency needs or aggressive impulses was blocked, the individual faced the risk for various physical illnesses. It was hypothesized that unexpressed dependency needs would lead to persistent stimulation of the parasympathetic nervous system, which, in turn, would increase the likelihood that the person might develop disorders such as ulcers, colitis, and asthma.

Historically, the concept of dependency has been of interest to social psychologists as well as to clinical psychologists, as social researchers have conducted many studies focusing on the relationship of dependency to interpersonal perceptions, beliefs, and behaviors. For instance, social dependence has been defined as a situation where some other person controls or possesses resources that the dependent person sees as necessary for him- or herself (Strong et al., 1992).

Much like clinical psychologists, social psychologists tend to regard dependency primarily in negative terms, viewing the dependent person as mainly interested in avoiding responsibility and interpersonal conflict. In exchange for their sense of helplessness, dependent persons try to compensate by occupying a lower status or a follower position.

Development and Causes

The cause of DPD is not known, but it is believed to be a combination of biological and developmental factors. For instance, people exposed to authoritarian or overprotective parents, chronic physical illness, or separation anxiety during childhood seem to be more likely to develop dependent personality traits. In comparing DPD to other personality disorders, some opinions indicate that DPD appears to be more environmentally influenced (Bjornlund, 2011). However, a 2012 study estimated that between 55 percent and 72 percent of the risk of the condition is inherited from one's parents (Gjerde et al., 2012).

Socialization practices regarding the expression of dependency needs vary among different cultures according to gender differences. For instance, it has been noted that dependency in adults seems to indicate a level of immaturity (Ainsworth, 1969). Other assertions regard dependency as devalued and pathologized and to be "linked with symbiosis, weakness, passivity, immaturity and is attributed to women, children, and persons perceived as inadequately functioning" (Siegel, 1988, p. 113). However, in other countries, such as Japan and India, both boys and girls are encouraged to express dependency needs openly (Kobayashi, 1989; Bloom, 1982).

Parenting behaviors and attitudes characterized by overprotectiveness and authoritarianism tend to result in an increase of dependent traits in their children. These parenting traits can limit the children from developing a sense of autonomy while teaching them that others are powerful and competent (Simonelli & Parolin, 2017). It is important to note that in general, parental behavior patterns such as permissiveness, conformity, overprotectiveness, and authoritarianism, as well as abusiveness and neglect, are associated with reinforcement of passive, dependent behavior in children and with the discouragement of independent, autonomous functioning.

On the other hand, just as parental overprotectiveness and authoritarianism can prevent children's trial-and-error learning that is so important for the development of their sense of self-confidence, so can parents' unrealistic independence and achievement expectations result in the child's continuing to exhibit high levels of passive-dependent behavior through the middle and late childhood years.

Studies assessing the relationship between dependency and popularity in schoolchildren have produced highly consistent results. In every study, dependency was associated with a lack of popularity and social acceptance by the dependent child's peers (Bornstein, 1993). So it would appear that once the dependency roots have been established in the child's home environment, they are likely to continue through the years of school and beyond.

Traits related to DPD, like most personality disorders, emerge in childhood. Findings from the NESARC study indicated that 18- to 29-year-old individuals have a greater chance of developing DPD. Children and adolescents with a history of physical illnesses and anxiety disorders seem to be more susceptible to acquiring DPD (Nolen-Hoeksema, 2014).

Individuals who experience traumatic events early in life, such as neglect and abuse or serious illness, can have an increased likelihood of developing personality disorders, including DPD, later in life. This is especially prevalent for those individuals who also experience great interpersonal stress and poor social support (Simonelli & Parolin, 2017).

As suggested by a 2004 twin study, there is a heritability of 0.81 percent for developing DPD. This is regarded as significant evidence that this disorder runs in families (Coolidge, Thede, & Jang, 2014).

Effects and Costs

Excessive dependence on others renders a person with DPD susceptible to experiencing additional problems, such as depression, bipolar disorder, panic disorder, generalized anxiety disorder, bulimia, and social phobia. The pessimism and lack of self-confidence experienced by people with DPD keeps them from making decisions in their own best interest and setting and achieving goals other than to be taken care of. In their intimate relationships, individuals with DPD will leave major decisions to their partners due to their fear of displeasing them and being abandoned by them. This will prevent them from achieving the fulfillment of their own goals and wishes. In their role as parents, people with DPD will most likely fail to be inspiring, self-confident, and competent examples for their children, and the risk of passing on their distressing condition to their children is significant as children tend to copy their parents' behaviors, and they may incorporate the parents' inability to function adequately without the help of others into their own personalities.

Furthermore, the fear of being alone and abandoned leaves those with DPD at risk of entering into and remaining in physically and/or mentally abusive relationships due to their willingness to tolerate mistreatment from others rather than be abandoned by them. Furthermore, an increased risk of suicide has been found among people with dependent personality disorder (Chioqueta & Stiles, 2004).

As has been demonstrated in many correlational studies assessing the relationship between individuals' dependency needs and the presence of depression, there is a significant positive relationship between levels of dependency and levels of depression. Thus, in addition to struggling with the effects of DPD, sufferers may experience the additional pain associated with depression.

Furthermore, psychoanalytic theory hypothesizes that dependency needs should be associated with a risk for obesity and a risk for eating disorders because dependent individuals tend to rely on "oral" activities to cope with the anxiety related to unfulfilled dependency needs.

Observations regarding the relationship of dependency to interpersonal sensitivity seem to indicate that as a group, dependent individuals tend to be highly skilled at decoding subtle interpersonal cues (Masling, Schiffner, & Shenfeld, 1980). Because the dependent person's "core" motivation is to obtain and maintain nurturant, supportive relationships, good social skills should be associated with success in finding supportive, helpful protectors. But, in turn, the presence of these protective supporters recapitulate for the dependent person the earlier parent-child relationship that led to the dependency in the first place. Thus, the mere presence of the new nurturant protector serves to reinforce the dependent person's "helpless" self-concept. And, as the dependent person with less effective social skills will be less successful in obtaining supportive, protective relationships, this in turn will lead to increased anxiety and stress.

In Society

Social relations tend to be limited to those few people on whom the individual is dependent. Any criticism and disapproval of people with DPD will be taken as proof of their worthlessness, and they lose faith in themselves and become even more dependent on others.

As individuals with DPD generally avoid taking on adult responsibilities by acting passive and helpless, their social interactions will usually occur while in the company of a spouse or friend. Otherwise, they might be a shadow at the periphery of a gathering or attempting to find a "rescuer" to hold on to. Others may feel uncomfortable in the presence of those afflicted with DPD because their avoidance of expressing an opinion (for fear of losing the support and approval of those around them) leaves others with the impression they don't really know the person with DPD.

The dependent behaviors of people with DPD occur consistently across different situations and settings, leading social perceivers to attribute the dependent behaviors to internal (dispositional) rather than to external (situational) cues. And even in situations where an individual's dependent behavior is clearly caused by the event, perceivers will most likely infer that the behavior reflects the person's underlying dependency needs. Therefore, regardless of the situation, the dependent person will be viewed and treated by others in terms of the person's "obvious" dependency needs. Their easily recognizable dependency needs become a social cue by which to recognize individuals with DPD.

Rather than risk losing the help of those to whom they look for guidance, dependent individuals' inability to function independently will lead them to agree with things or situations that they feel are wrong. The consequences could be costly.

Up Close
When it came time to apply for college, Amanda was at a loss. Most of her friends and classmates had already made their choices and applied

to various colleges in different states. But Amanda could not conceive of leaving home. How would she be able to take care of her needs? How would she decide what outfits to wear to different occasions? All her young life, she had relied on her mother and older sister, Eva, to guide her in those matters. As Eva married her boyfriend soon after graduation from high school, Amanda could not count on her sister for advice at college away from home. But Eva suggested that Amanda attend a local community college for the next two years to prevent the need for out-of-state tuition costs. As usual, Amanda was grateful to Eva for her guidance. It was difficult enough to get used to a new educational environment; at least she did not have to worry about having to live with strangers, and she still had the help and guidance of her family.

Two years later, after graduation from community college, Amanda's anxiety rose to an unbearable level; she faced the same problem: how could she function away from home? Again, Eva, a mother by now, had the solution. Amanda could apply at the local hospital for health care–related training. Again, Amanda followed Eva's advice and became increasingly more dependent on her. What would she do without her older sister? Amanda asked herself. "Never leave her" was the obvious answer. Again, her fears of leaving her home environment were reinforced, and she became a reliable employee at the hospital. In her free time, Amanda helped her aging parents and spent time with Eva and her growing family.

During adolescence, Amanda had discovered that eating helped her cope with the increasing anxiety she experienced in any situation that involved change or interactions with others except immediate family members. As her body size increased, her chances of dating any of the local boys and young men decreased. Even girlfriends seemed to have less time to spend with Amanda. She feared that they did not want to be seen with her, but she never confronted them about it; it was just too embarrassing. Her increasing obesity made Amanda even more dependent on her family. Her bouts with depression were dealt with through the use of medication, easily obtained from some of the hospital's physicians. When Amanda's mother died, leaving Amanda with her father in the family home, Amanda was at a loss about assuming responsibility for him and herself. She expressed suicidal ideation to the physician who provided the antidepressant medication. He, in turn, with Amanda's permission, communicated with Eva, who by now was the mother of three lively children. During the family discussion, the decision was reached to sell the old family home and add two bedrooms and a bathroom to Eva's current home to accommodate Amanda and their father. Thus,

Amanda's life became even more intertwined with her family's life, leaving no need for additional relationships except those of a superficial nature within her job environment.

At Work

Many individuals with DPD will not begin tasks, because they believe others could probably do better with those tasks. Even if they have the ability to carry out a job, rather than perform the job activities independently, they will often present themselves as inept. And by avoiding challenges, they give up opportunities to learn more (Bayer, 2000). Their difficulty with initiating projects or doing things on their own is due not so much to a lack of motivation or energy but rather because of a lack of self-confidence in their own judgment or abilities. Desperately wanting the support of others, individuals with DPD will often volunteer to do things (job tasks) that are unpleasant.

These individuals, feeling incapable of making decisions, may rely on others, such as parents, in their contemplations what types of jobs to apply and/or train for, with the result of entering employment they don't actually enjoy. And at times being unable to even make simple decisions, such as whether or not to take an umbrella along or what to wear, they may encounter difficulties making decisions about their job-related wardrobe.

Of interest in work settings may be the results found when a peer rather than a figure of authority functioned as experimenter in a verbal conditioning study; an effect of dependency on responsiveness to verbal reinforcement was obtained. As observed in other research, dependent individuals are more responsive to figures of authority than peers in verbal conditioning experiments (Cooperman & Child, 1971).

Up Close
As the youngest of three brothers, Richard had always been dependent on his brothers for most decisions, such as what sports to participate in, what teachers to like through his school years, even what types of clothes and shoes to wear. His brothers had the answers to everything— or so it seemed. In his senior year in high school, he even dated Joyce, the younger sister of the girl his next older brother dated. Even though his brothers teased him about wanting to be part of all their activities, Richard swallowed his hurt feelings and insisted on hanging onto them. Although Joyce agreed to be his prom date, she broke up with Richard soon after that because of his clinging behavior. And, as she said,

their relationship was going to end anyway because she was planning to attend college in a different state. Richard was heartbroken and clung even tighter to his brothers.

He did not apply to any college, not even being sure of what his future work life should look like. In the meantime, his oldest brother, Anthony, had joined a local construction firm. What better opportunity for Richard than to join his brother's workplace? He was permitted to work under his brother's close supervision. Richard was grateful and followed his brother's every decision and order. Having his brother take on the responsibility for Richard's performance seemed to assure Richard's future life situation.

Anthony was ambitious and planned to have his own construction company some day. He shared some of his dreams with Richard and promised him that there would always be a place for Richard as long as he remained loyal to Anthony.

Anthony, newly married and soon to be a father, had started on the creation of his new home. It occurred to him that some of the company's materials seemed perfect for his future home. He enlisted Richard's help in appropriating various of the company's building materials. Richard was shocked; this was theft! But if Anthony needed those materials, Richard had to make sure he got them. He could not let his brother down; besides, Anthony would get him fired and abandon him if he did not do what was expected of him. Richard could not conceive of a life without Anthony's guidance and support. Choosing between the loyalty he owed his employer, the construction company, and the risk of abandonment by his brother, Richard sacrificed his obligations and responsibility to his employer.

In Relationships

Although individuals with DPD try hard to please others, they often do not have close, satisfying relationships in which their own needs are met (Overholser, 1996). As stated earlier, individuals with DPD, with their dependency on others, tend to have difficulty making the best decisions for themselves because of their fear of losing the approval of those around them. As part of their dependency, they tend to place the needs and opinions of others above their own and engage in passive and clingy behavior, which in long-term relationships can lead to stressful interactions.

In addition, people with DPD are often pessimistic in their outlook on life. They tend to expect the worst out of situations and steadfastly hold onto the belief that the worst will happen. This pessimistic attitude can destroy the overall mood in close relationships (Beitz, 2006).

Some researchers have hypothesized that in romantic relationships, dependency would be associated with increased commitment because the dependent person is very much concerned with maintaining close ties to supportive, nurturing figures (Simpson & Gangestad, 1991). On the other hand, if an important relationship ends, desperation to fill the void overwhelms dependent personalities. They are frantic to find a new friend or lover and often don't choose carefully enough—and, hence, end up in a disastrous new relationship. Because of their intense fear of abandonment, individuals with DPD often show a willingness to tolerate mistreatment and abuse from others (Cleveland Clinic News and More, 2017). On the other hand, their need for care and support can lead to abusive behavior, intimidation, and violence in some men. This kind of dependency may be reflected by a jealous man who abuses his wife or partner. Dependent men are at risk of becoming abusers when fearing that the partner is about to leave.

Thus, within relationships, dependency can be a risk factor for abusive behavior in at least two ways. One of the risk factors reflects the "social cue" aspect of dependency, such as dependency exhibited by a nonworking spouse, while the other risk factor is connected to the dependency needs of a potential abuser. In this way, both "provider" and "providee" dependency may be involved in child, parental, and spousal abuse (Bornstein, 1993).

Up Close

Growing up loved and protected by her parents and older brother, Cynthia was not used to making decisions or assuming responsibilities for more than her school attendance and which friends to play with. Her father was a self-made business owner who enjoyed spoiling his family with the rewards from his business. "What else is money for if not to make your family happy?" he used to say. Cynthia's mother was pleased with her husband's position as the kind, generous head of the family. Greg, the oldest child, was expected to take over the family business when his father was ready to retire, and, as would be expected, he had a close relationship with his father.

Although not ambitious, Cynthia kept up with her schoolwork. She always sat next to the same friends and was rarely seen alone. Cynthia's toys resembled those of her friends, and so did her clothes. It was one of Cynthia's ways to avoid expressing disagreement.

Cynthia's father jokingly described his family as consisting of two beauties and two brains, with Cynthia's mother and Cynthia being the beauties.

When it came time for Cynthia to think about her professional future, her mother suggested that she become a dental hygienist, which would allow her to change her schedule to accommodate her changing family needs. This sounded like good advice as Cynthia had started dating Mark, her brother's best friend.

Mark adored Cynthia, and during their marriage, he treated her in many ways like her father and brother had done. Cynthia found employment at a local dental office, and the young couple prepared to start a family. Cynthia was two months pregnant when Mark died in an automobile accident on his way home from a business trip.

Cynthia was crushed. She could not move back in with her parents, because they had already made commitments to move into a retirement community in Florida. Greg, her brother, had married, and he and his wife promised to help Cynthia in her grief and adjustment to becoming a single mother.

Through her work Cynthia met Harold, a pharmaceutical representative who paid regular visits to the dental office and other medical clinics in the same office building. Harold was charming and attentive and convinced Cynthia that meeting for a cup of coffee would be good for both of them, as he still was working through some disappointment from his divorce. Their meetings increased in frequency, and Harold eventually disclosed that his feelings for Cynthia went deeper than friendship.

With her pregnancy progressing, Cynthia's anxiety about the responsibility of raising her child by herself increased. Harold proposed marriage, suggesting to Cynthia that it would be best for the child and Cynthia if they got married before the birth of the child, so that the child would have two parents from the beginning. Later, when the child was old enough to understand the situation, they would tell the child about the real father. Although shocked at first, Cynthia agreed with Harold's proposal as a solution to her problem.

In a quiet ceremony, Cynthia and Harold got married before Cynthia gave birth to her daughter. This marriage was different from her first marriage. Although—as before—her husband made all the decisions, Harold's personality was not as gentle as Mark's had been. Harold's basic belief that men were the rulers of their families was strengthened by the entitlement he felt for having saved Cynthia from the fate of being a single parent. Cynthia did not dare express disagreement. She tried her best to quietly fulfill Harold's expectations, but her increasing anxiety impaired the quality of her chores at home as well as her performance at her job. Harold's expressions of disappointment in Cynthia's performance became stronger over time and finally included physical punishment. Cynthia did not complain; she was afraid that Harold would leave her. She did not even tell Greg about the abuse until the day Harold beat her in front of her little daughter, who started screaming hysterically and would not stop.

Theory and Research

Psychodynamic theories suggest that unconscious emotional conflicts and the unconscious defenses against them shape individuals' personality traits. And it is thought that dependent personalities are defending themselves against unconscious hostility. They feel the need to ward off this emotion, which was originally directed against overbearing parents. As a result, these individuals submit to others as a way to avoid showing or even acknowledging anger.

Because the concept of dependency is of interest to researchers in many different areas, numerous measures of dependency have been developed since the late 1940s. Among the different measures, interpersonal dependency scales tend to utilize an objective format, requiring subjects to respond to direct questions regarding dependent thoughts, feelings, and behaviors. The test items in these scales consist of a series of self-statements, with the majority employing a true-false format, although a few of them use Likert-type ratings, asking subjects to declare which statements in particular test items apply to them. In general, objective interpersonal dependency measures have high face validity, meaning that they are obviously tapping dependency-related traits.

On the other hand, objective oral dependency measures, while utilizing the same self-statement format that the objective interpersonal dependency measures do, require subjects to respond to questions regarding preoccupation with food, eating, and other "oral" activities—because they are closely tied to psychoanalytic theory—in addition to questions concerned with dependent thoughts, feelings, and behaviors.

Both objective interpersonal and objective oral dependency scales yield several dependency-related subscale scores in addition to a global dependency score. Most of these subscales were developed using factor analysis or cluster analysis.

In contrast to objective dependency scales, projective dependency measures require individuals to respond to ambiguous stimuli, such as inkblots or drawings. Individuals' responses are scored by experimenters for either dependent or oral dependent content. The ambiguity inherent in projective dependency measures can be seen as a strength because subjects are not aware of the type of information the experimenter plans to draw from their responses. Their low face validity makes projective dependency measures relatively immune from self-report and self-representation biases. But there is a limitation. These scales generally provide only a single, global index of level of dependency. In addition, a number of interview and rating measures have been developed (Bornstein, 1993).

Regarding the epigenesis of dependency, studies can be divided into two areas. Several researchers have tested the psychoanalytic hypothesis that childhood, adolescent, and adult dependency can be traced to feeding and weaning experiences during infancy. Taking a somewhat broader view, other researchers have examined the relationship between various aspects of the parent-child relationship and later dependency.

One of the most important determinants of the specific form that dependency strivings will take in males and females has been determined to be sex-role socialization. Traditional sex-role socialization practices lead men to express dependency needs indirectly—often turning to physical violence—and lead women to express dependency needs in a more direct and overt manner.

The long-held assumption that women are more dependent than men may require a closer look. It appears that the likelihood that sex differences in dependency will surface in any given study is a function of the type of dependency measure used in that investigation. For example, it was found that when self-report measures of dependency are used, most studies examining gender differences in adult dependency resulted in significantly higher levels of dependency in women than in men. Schoolchildren also showed similar gender differences in dependency with self-report measures. However, with the use of projective measures of dependency, researchers typically find that men and women (and boys and girls) exhibit similar levels of dependency. These patterns were found in both nonclinical subjects and psychiatric patients (Bornstein, 1993).

As women in their self-reports seem to view themselves as more dependent than men, the intuitive suggestion might indicate a cultural basis, such as sex-role socialization. It is of interest that similar gender differences on self-report dependency measures are found in American, British, German, Japanese, and Indian subjects (Bornstein, 1993).

Studies that were assessing the relationship of dependency to sex-role orientation revealed results that clearly support the hypothesis that the overt expression of dependency needs in both men and women is a function of the degree to which individuals ascribe to traditional sex roles.

Among studies focusing on various personality dimensions that predict risk factors for physical illness, a correlation of .35 was found between level of dependency assessed at age 20 and global physical illness ratings obtained at age 50 (Vaillant, 1978). In general, research findings indicate that level of dependency is at least as strong a predictor of risk for physical illness as other theoretically related personality traits. Actually, dependency may be a better risk predictor for disease than other traits. But what is the mechanism by which dependency increases a person's risk for physical problems? Some hypotheses have focused on the likelihood that dependency—when coupled with events in the environment that activate feelings of helplessness and dependency—puts a person at risk for a variety of physical illnesses. In other words, a type of "relationship anxiety" may play a role in mediating the dependency-disease link (Greenberg & Bornstein, 1988).

Important implications for a dependency-affiliation relationship have emerged from a study involving 241 unmarried, monogamous couples. Each subject provided three pieces of information: a self-report of level of dependency, a rating of his or her commitment to the relationship, and an estimate of his or her partner's degree of commitment to the relationship. The findings from this investigation revealed that there was a significant positive correlation between level of dependency and degree of commitment to the relationship in both men and women. There was also a significant positive correlation between level of dependency and estimates of the partner's degree of commitment to the relationship in men and in women. This means that dependency is not only associated with increased commitment in romantic relationships, but also that level of dependency predicts subjects' perception of their partner's commitment to the relationship (Simpson & Gangestad, 1991).

The outcomes of studies concerned with the dependency-help-seeking relationship raised questions about how the behavior of dependent individuals might be affected when they are forced to work independently while knowing that their performance would be evaluated by authority figures. Experiments examining the relationship between dependency and performance anxiety in laboratory problem-solving situations and field studies investigating the relationship between dependency and academic performance revealed varying outcomes, but overall, they were consistent with the hypothesis that dependency is associated with high levels of performance anxiety in laboratory settings when subjects are required to work independently (Bornstein, 1993).

Focusing on dependency and academic performance, another study used a mixed sample of 107 10th graders and found a strong relationship between dependency and underachievement (Tesser & Blusiewicz, 1987).

Another aspect of dependency-related behavior of interest to researchers has been the link of dependency and treatment duration. Several studies have indicated that dependent individuals tend to remain in treatment longer than do nondependent individuals. The underlying presumption was that the dependent person is reluctant to give up the patient-caretaker relationship. The effects of patient dependency to treatment duration were statistically significant as long as the treatment consisted of inpatient treatment at hospitals; but studies of the dependency-treatment duration relationship in outpatients have yielded more mixed, inconclusive findings (Bornstein, 1993).

It should be noted here that research on the developmental, social, and clinical aspects of dependency has examined the effects of exaggerated dependency needs on some *other* dimension of behavior and thereby differs from research focusing on dependent personality disorder where most studies are concerned with the prevalence of DPD in various subject groups, on the relationship of DPD to other psychological disorders, and on the reliability of DPD symptoms and diagnoses.

Of interest regarding the theoretical basis of DPD is the *Psychodynamic Diagnostic Manual* (PDM), which approaches DPD in a descriptive, rather than prescriptive, sense. The *PDM* distinguishes between two different types of dependent personality disorder: the passive-aggressive and the counter-dependent types (Simonelli & Parolin, 2017).

The *PDM-2* follows a prototypic approach, using empirical measures like the SWAP 200, a diagnostic tool developed with the goal of overcoming certain limitations. In the context of the SWAP-200, DPD is considered a clinical prototype rather than discrete symptoms, and it provides composite description characteristic criteria, such as personality tendencies (Simonelli & Parolin, 2017). The PDM-2 approach was influenced by a developmental and empirically grounded perspective and is of particular interest when focusing on DPD, claiming that psychopathology arises from distortions of two main coordinates of psychological development, namely, the anaclitic/introjective and the relatedness/self-definition dimensions (Simonelli & Parolin, 2017). The anaclitic personality organization in individuals exhibits difficulties in interpersonal relatedness, whereas the introjective personality style is associated with problems in self-definition (Simonelli & Parolin, 2017).

According to behavioral and social learning theory, two kinds of learning—conditioning and reinforcement—function in children's development of habits that constitute personality. Based on this model, children who are rewarded for making excessive demands for care may develop a dependent personality. Parents who are inconsistent may leave children with the lesson that they cannot control their own lives.

Cognitive psychology explains dependency as a result of the way people think about themselves and others. Dependent personalities tell themselves that they are powerless, facing others who are powerful. A study of psychiatric outpatients investigating the relationship within Cluster C personality disorders and suicide attempts found that only DPD was associated with suicide attempts (Chioqueta & Stiles, 2004).

Studies have reported strong relationships between people with DPD and alcohol and drug problems, especially for men (Grant et al., 2004). And over 50 percent of people with DPD showed comorbidity with avoidant, obsessive-compulsive and/or borderline personality disorders, according to a 2010 study (Bjornlund, 2011).

Signs of dependent personality can be observed in brief encounters with strangers, according to a 2006 experiment. Nearly 100 women, half of them psychology students and half of them recruited through an advertisement, were asked to participate in improvised skits confronting a waitress who had served the wrong order, a friend asking for a personal loan, and a persistent door-to-door salesman. Observers, asked to judge the women on how well they stood up for themselves, noted that both dependent and avoidant personality traits were linked to low assertiveness, but for different reasons. Women with dependent traits were afraid they would not be liked, whereas the women with avoidant personality traits regarded their own needs as unimportant (Leising, Sporberg, & Rehbein, 2006).

Some types of personality disorders appear more vulnerable to being victims of violence, as shown in a 2009 study. Researchers were exploring whether people with DPD were at greater risk of being abused by their spouse. They worked with a sample of 305 participants receiving outpatient services for physical abuse and found that, indeed, people with DPD suffered spousal abuse more often than people with other personality disorders or people with no personality disorder (Bjornlund, 2011). But despite what has generally been assumed, studies have not revealed a high rate of dependent personality among abused women. Although many of these women exhibited dependent traits, it was mainly due to their being terrorized, isolated, economically dependent, or worried about their children. However, when considering the most severely abused women as a separate group, there is some evidence that dependent personality is more common. This may be because such women are more vulnerable to begin with, or they may find it more difficult to leave even when that would be the best choice for them (Harvard Mental Health Letter, 2007).

Psychologist Theodore Millon conceived of five adult subtypes of dependent personality disorder. According to this classification, any dependent individual may exhibit none or one of the following subtypes: disquieted-dependent, selfless-dependent, immature-dependent, accommodating-dependent, and ineffectual-dependent. In their various descriptions, the subtypes appear to share features of other personality disorders. For instance, the disquieted-dependent subtype includes avoidant features, while the accommodating-dependent subtype includes histrionic features, and the ineffectual-dependent subtype is thought to share features with schizoid personality disorder (Millon, 2006).

There are also similarities between individuals with DPD and those with borderline personality disorder, as both exhibit a fear of abandonment (Murphy & Cowan, 2009).

Treatment

Many people with DPD do not seek out treatment, and those who do will wait until the disorder starts to significantly interfere with their daily lives. Usually that happens when the person's coping resources are stretched too thin to handle any stressful situations (Bressert, 2017). Generally, people with DPD are treated with psychotherapy with the main goal of making individuals more independent and assist them in forming healthy relationships with the people around them. This usually requires improvement of the individuals' self-esteem and confidence.

Various types of psychotherapy are of help for this condition. In psychodynamic therapy, patients are led to explore past relationships that fostered dependent behavior, and they learn to understand how these are reflected in internalized images of themselves and others, including the therapist. Cognitive therapy is helpful in focusing on the patient's thinking patterns, exposing and correcting unrealistic judgments based on false underlying beliefs. Behavioral therapy would address the patient's behavior patterns, trying to alter cause-effect relationships and incentives that promote compulsive care-seeking—all meant to help individuals gain greater assertiveness and social skills. During the beginning stages of therapy, patients may try to shift all responsibility for decisions and changes to the therapist. Joint therapy with family members can also be helpful in resolving relational problems.

Recovery for any disorder depends on changing entrenched attitudes and behaviors, and people often feel worse before they feel better. Some disorders seem to be more resistant to treatment than others, and research indicates that the elements of DPD may be particularly resistant to change because human interdependence generally continues throughout life for most. The goal of therapy is to reduce the exaggerated level of helplessness that individuals with DPD exhibit. A therapist may be able to help individuals just enough so that a personality disorder turns into a personality type—polite, agreeable, respectful of others and their opinions, disliking solitude, and preferring to be a follower rather than a leader.

Medication is not necessarily used as a primary treatment for DPD, but antidepressants, sedatives, and tranquilizers may be used in conjunction with other psychiatric conditions, such as depression and anxiety disorder, but it does not treat the core problems caused by DPD.

References

Ainsworth, M. D. S. (1969). Object relations, dependency and attachment: A theoretical review of the infant-mother relationship. *Child Development, 40*, 969–1025.

Alexander, F. (1950). *Psychosomatic medicine*. New York, NY: W. W. Norton.

Bayer, L. (2000). *Personality disorders*. Philadelphia, PA: Chelsea House Publishers.

Beitz, K. (2006). *Dependent personality disorder (Practitioner's guide to evidence-based psychotherapy)*. Boston, MA: Springer.

Bjornlund, L. (2011). *Personality disorders*. San Diego, CA: Reference Point Press.

Bloom, L. (1982). Socialization and dependence in Nigeria. *Journal of Social Psychology, 117*, 3–12.

Bornstein, R. F. (1993). *The dependent personality*. New York, NY: The Guilford Press.

Bornstein, R. F. (1996). Sex differences in dependent personality disorder prevalence rates. *Clinical Psychology: Science and Practice, 3*(1). doi:10.1111/j.1468-2850.1996.tb00054.x

Bressert, S. (2017). Dependent personality disorder symptoms. *Psych Central*. Retrieved February 2, 2018, from https://psychcentral.com /disorders/dependent-personality-disorder/symptoms/

Chioqueta, A. P., & Stiles, T. C. (2004). Assessing suicide risk in Cluster C personality disorders. *Crisis, 25*(3), 128–133.

Cleveland Clinic News and More. (2017). Dependent personality disorder. *Cleveland Clinic.* Retrieved from https://my.clevelandclinic.org/health/diseases/9783-dependent-personality-disorder

Coolidge, F. L., Thede, L., & Jang, K. L. (2004). Are personality disorders psychological manifestations of executive function deficits? Bivariate heritability evidence from a twin study. *Behavior Genetics, 34,* 75–84.

Cooperman, M., & Child, I. (1971). Differential effects of positive and negative reinforcement on two psychoanalytic character types. *Journal of Consulting and Clinical Psychology, 37,* 57–59.

Gjerde, L. C., Czajkowski, N., Roysamb, E., Orstavik, R. E., Knudsen, G. P., Ostby, K., . . . , Reichborn-Kjennerud, T. (2012). The heritability of avoidant and dependent personality disorder assessed by personal interview and questionnaire. *Acta Psychiatrica Scandinavica, 128*(6), 448–457.

Grant, B. F., Stinson, F. S., Dawson, D. A., Chou, S. P., Ruan, W. J., & Pickering, R. P. (2004). Co-occurrence of 12-month alcohol and drug use disorders and personality disorders in the United States: Results from the National Epidemiologic Survey on Alcohol and related conditions. *Archives of General Psychiatry, 61*(4), 361–368.

Greenberg, R. P., & Bornstein, R. F. (1988). The dependent personality, I: Risk for physical disorders. *Journal of Personality Disorders, 2,* 126–135.

Harvard Mental Health Letter. (April 2007). *Dependent personality disorder.* Boston, MA: Harvard Health Publishing. Harvard Medical School.

Leising, D., Sporberg, D., & Rehbein, D. (2006). Characteristic interpersonal behavior in dependent and avoidant personality disorder can be observed within very short interaction sequences. *Journal of Personality Disorders, 20*(4), 319–330.

Masling, J. M., Schiffner, J., & Shenfeld, M. (1980). Client perception of the therapist, orality, and sex of client and therapist. *Journal of Counseling Psychology, 27,* 294–298.

Millon, T. (2006). Millon Clinical Multiaxial Inventory III (MCMI-III) manual, 3rd ed. Minneapolis, MN: Pearson Assessments. Personality subtypes. Retrieved from http://millon.net/taxonomy/summary.htm

Murphy, M., & Cowan, R. (2009). *Blueprints psychiatry.* Philadelphia, PA: Lippincott Williams & Wilkins.

Nolen-Hoeksema, S. (2014). *Abnormal psychology* (6th ed.). New York, NY: McGraw Hill Education.

Overholser, J. C. (1996). The dependent personality and interpersonal problems. *Journal of Nervous and Mental Disease, 184*(1), 8–16.

Siegel, R. J. (1988). Women's dependency in a male-centered value system. *Women and Therapy, 7,* 113–133.

Simonelli, A., & Parolin, M. (2017). *Encyclopedia of personality and individual differences* (pp. 1–11). New York, NY: Springer.

Simpson, J. A., & Gangestad, W. W. (1991). Individual differences in sociosexuality: Evidence for convergent and discriminant validity. *Journal of Personality and Social Psychology, 60,* 870–883.

Strong, S. R., Welsh, J. A., Corcoran, J. L., & Hoyt, W. T. (1992). Social psychology and counseling psychology: The history, products and promise of an interface. *Journal of Counseling Psychology, 39,* 139–157.

Tesser, A., & Blusiewicz, C. O. (1987). Dependency conflict and underachievement. *Journal of Social and Clinical Psychology, 5,* 378–390.

Torgersen, S., Kringlen, E., & Cramer, V. (2001). The prevalence of personality disorders in a community sample. *Archives of General Psychiatry, 58*(6), 590–596.

Vaillant, G. E. (1978). Natural history of male psychological health, IV: What kinds of men do not get psychosomatic illness? *Psychosomatic Medicine, 40,* 420–431.

CHAPTER 5

Histrionic Personality Disorder

Symptoms, Diagnosis, and Incidence

Histrionic personality disorder (HPD) lies in the dramatic cluster of personality disorders. Its essential feature is a pervasive and excessive emotionality and attention-seeking behavior, a pattern that starts in early adulthood and is present in a variety of contexts.

People with HPD often exhibit lively, dramatic behaviors in order to draw attention to themselves because they feel unappreciated and uncomfortable when they are not the center of attention. Initially they may charm new acquaintances with their enthusiasm or flirtatiousness, but with their continuous demand for attention, those qualities lose their charm over time. In clinical settings, these individuals may provide dramatic descriptions of their physical and psychological symptoms, they might bring gifts for the clinician, and overall exhibit flattering behaviors. Their general appearance and behavior may often be sexually provocative or seductive, not only when interacting with persons they may have a romantic interest in but also in a wide variety of interactions within social, occupational, and professional relationships. Individuals with this disorder are overly concerned with their appearance and expend excessive amounts of energy and money on clothes and grooming—all with the goal to impress others with their appearance. It has been observed that as they age, some people with HPD change their seduction techniques to more maternal or paternal styles (Arthur, 2010).

The speech of those afflicted with HPD is often excessively impressionistic without regard to detail. Though they express strong opinions with dramatic flair, the underlying reasons may remain vague and diffuse, lacking supporting facts and details in the emotionally exaggerated comments of those with HPD. Their excessive public displays of emotion may become sources of embarrassment for friends and acquaintances. But despite the excessive display, their emotions often appear to be turned on and off too quickly to be deeply felt.

As individuals with HPD have a high degree of suggestibility, their opinions and feelings are easily influenced by others and by current trends or fads. Furthermore, they may be overly trusting, especially in those who seem to be in a position to help them solve their problems. They also often tend to regard relationships with others to be more intimate than they really are.

The prevalence of HPD, based on data from the 2001–2002 National Epidemiologic Survey on Alcohol and Related Conditions, has been estimated to be 1.84 percent. Other estimates range from 1–3 percent to 2–3 percent within the general population, with about equal probability among men and women. However, the way the characteristic traits are expressed may vary depending on the person's gender. For instance, men with HPD may brag incessantly about their golf scores, while women may express emotions in an excessive manner or dramatize themselves by wearing the latest fashions (Bayer, 2000).

Although this disorder has been diagnosed more frequently in females than in males in clinical settings, the sex ratio apparently is not significantly different from the sex ratio of females to males within the respective clinical setting. Yet other estimates state that typically at least two-thirds of persons with HPD are female, although there are some exceptions (Corbitt & Widiger, 1995). Other estimates indicate that HPD is diagnosed four times as frequently in women as in men (Seligman, 1984).

An estimated prevalence of 65 percent of HPD diagnoses in women compared to 35 percent in men elicited the response that women are generally over diagnosed due to potential biases to the point that even healthy women are often automatically diagnosed with HPD (Kaplan, 1983). Another explanation for the over-diagnosing of HPD in women may be that attention seeking and flirtation or sexual forwardness, traits expressed by people with HPD, are less socially acceptable for women than for men (Psychology Today, 2018).

It has been stated that HPD, while being associated with a distorted self-image, is the only personality disorder to be explicitly related to physical appearance (Kandola, 2017). Apparently, 10 to 15 percent of those in substance abuse treatment settings have HPD. HPD has been associated with alcoholism and with higher rates of somatization disorder, conversion disorder, and major depressive disorder as well as with other personality disorders, such as borderline, narcissistic, antisocial, and dependent personality disorders.

Timeline

1900 BC	First description of the mental disorder in Ancient Egypt.
5th century BC	Hippocrates was the first to use the term *hysteria*.
12th century	Trota of Salerno, a female medical practitioner, included hysteria in the texts of the *Trotula*.
17th century	Thomas Willis introduces a new concept of hysteria.
18th century	Franz Mesmer treated patients suffering from hysteria with his method, called mesmerism (or animal magnetism).
19th century	Jean-Martin Charcot studied effects of hypnosis in hysteria.
Late 19th century	Sigmund Freud studied histrionic personality disorder in a psychological manner.

History

The word histrionic means "dramatic" or "theatrical" or "hysterical." Similar to ancient Egyptians, the ancient Greeks saw hysteria being related to the uterus. Biological issues, such as the uterus movement in the female body, were thought to be the cause of hysteria. Traditional symptoms of hysteria are described in the Ebers Papyrus, the oldest medical document.

Hippocrates believed hysteria was a disease within the movement of the uterus. His theory that the uterus was prone to illness was based on women's bodies being cold and wet compared to men's bodies, which are warm and dry. This illness would happen to women especially when they were deprived of sex. Hippocrates saw sex as the cleansing of the body; overemotionality was due to sex deprivation.

In the 12th century, Trota of Salerno, a female medical practitioner responsible for the texts of the *Trotula* discussing women's diseases and disorders, including hysteria, as understood during this time period.

During the Renaissance, the uterus was still used as explanation of hysteria, and the concept of women's inferiority to men was still present. Hysteria continued to be the symbol for femininity (Tasca, Rapetti, Carta, & Fadda, 2012).

In the 17th century, Thomas Willis believed that the causes of hysteria were not linked to the uterus of the female but rather to the brain and nervous system. During the Age of Enlightenment (17th to 18th century), the notion of hysteria was developed in a more scientific way, especially neurologically. One of the new ideas formed during this time was that hysteria is connected to the brain, and men could possess it, too, not just women.

Charcot regarded hysteria as a neurological disease that is actually quite common in men. *Studies on Hysteria*, the work of Sigmund Freud and Josef Breuer, was a contribution to a psychoanalytic theory of hysteria, suggesting that hysteria was caused by a lack of libidinal evolution (Tasca et al., 2012).

The results of Freud's development of psychoanalytic theory led to split concepts of hysteria. One concept was labeled "hysterical neurosis" (also known as conversion disorder), and the other concept was called "hysterical character" (currently known as histrionic personality disorder). These two concepts represent two separate and different ideas and should not be confused with each other (Pfohl, 1994).

Hysterical personality, another name for HPD, has evolved in the past 400 years (Alam & Merskey, 1992). It first appeared in the *DSM-II* under the name *hysterical personality disorder*. The change to the current name, histrionic personality disorder, occurred in *DSM-III*, apparently because of possible negative connotations to the roots of hysteria, such as intense sexual expressions, demon possessions, and other similar characteristics (Bakkevig & Sigmund, 2010).

HPD has gone through many changes. As one of the oldest documented medical disorders, hysteria in most of the writings has been related to women, similar to today, where the epidemiology of HPD is more prevalent in women and also more frequently diagnosed in women (Sutker, 2002).

The overdiagnosing of women with this disorder is largely due to Western culture. If men are bragging about their accomplishments, it is considered to be part of being macho; but if a woman seeks the same kind of attention, she most likely will be diagnosed with histrionic personality disorder (Lumen Learning, 2018).

Theodore Millon has identified six subtypes of histrionic personality disorder: the appeasing, the vivacious, the tempestuous, the disingenuous, the theatrical, and the infantile histrionic (Millon, 2004). Some of the subtypes seem to include characteristics from other disorders.

Because of the apparent prevalence of histrionic personality disorder in women, recommendations for re-evaluation of culturally constructed ideas around what is considered normal emotional behavior have been made. The diagnostic approach classifies the behaviors of histrionic personality disorder as "excessive," considering it in reference to a social understanding of normal emotionality (American Psychiatric Association).

The use of a mnemonic to remember the characteristics of histrionic personality disorder has been suggested (Pinkofsky, 1997), with the shortened phrase "PRAISE ME" representing the following traits: Provocative (or seductive) behavior. Relationships are considered more intimate than they actually are. Attention seeking. Influenced easily by others or circumstances. Speech (style) wants to impress; lacks detail. Emotional lability; shallowness. Makeup; physical appearance is used to draw attention to self. Exaggerated emotions; theatrical.

Development and Causes

In psychoanalytic theory, a series of psychosexual stages of development determines an individual's later psychological development. According to early psychoanalysts, the genital phase, Freud's fifth or last stage of psychosexual development, was thought to be a determinant of HPD. But later psychoanalysts viewed the oral phase, Freud's first stage of psychosexual development, as a more important determinant of HPD. There is agreement among most psychoanalysts that a traumatic childhood contributes to the development of HPD. Some theorists suggest that disapproval in the early mother-child relationship may result in more severe HPD cases.

Freud's theory also suggests that people use various defense mechanisms to cope with conflict and reduce anxiety. In the case of individuals with HPD, the severity of the maladaptive defense mechanisms differs with the severity of the disorder. For instance, patients with more severe impairment may use the defense mechanisms of repression, denial, and even dissociation (Lumen Learning, 2018).

Social and biological factors contribute to the development of personality, according to biosocial models in psychology and biosocial learning models. They suggest that individuals may develop HPD as a result of inconsistent interpersonal reinforcement offered by parents; for example, individuals with HPD may have learned to get what they want from others by drawing attention to themselves.

Studies of specific cultures having high rates of HPD would suggest social and cultural causes of HPD.

Many mental health professionals believe that both learned and inherited factors have an impact on the development of HPD. A genetic susceptibility for the disorder is indicated by the tendency to run in families. However, it may also be that the child of a parent with HPD is just repeating learned behavior. Other environmental factors involved in a particular case might include a lack of criticism or punishment when a child misbehaves. Furthermore, unpredictable parental attention may lead to confusion in the child's mind about what types of behavior are acceptable and which ones are unacceptable (WebMD, 2018).

The development of HPD may reflect a complicated interaction of biological predisposition and environmental responses. The traits of extroversion and emotional expressiveness, which are basic to the character of individuals with HPD, are recognized as having biological components. It is thought that these factors interact with a lack of caregiver attention during the child's formative years and eventually lead to the development of attention-grabbing strategies and shallow interaction that would elicit attention and connection (Lumen Learning, 2018).

Some family history studies have observed that histrionic personality disorder as well as borderline and antisocial personality disorders tend to run in families, although it is not clear whether this is due to genetic or environmental factors. A predisposition could be a factor as to why some people are diagnosed with HPD. It is not known, however, whether or not the disorder is influenced by any biological compound or is genetically inheritable (Nolen-Hoeksema, 2014).

In psychoanalytic theory, authoritarian or distant parental attitudes (mainly the mother), along with conditional love based on expectations the child can never fulfill, are thought to be the precipitating factors (Bienenfeld, 2006). It was Freud's belief that lustfulness was a projection of an individual's lack of ability to love unconditionally and to develop mentally to maturity, leaving such individuals emotionally shallow (Pfohl, 1995). Traumatic experiences, such as the death of a close relative during childhood or divorce of one's parents, might be reasons for the inability to love.

Most people with HPD also have other mental disorders, such as antisocial, dependent, borderline, and narcissistic personality disorders (Hales & Yudofski, 2003), as well as depression, anxiety, panic, and somatoform disorders, including attachment disorder.

HPD usually begins by the late teens or early 20s. In the beginning stages of this disorder, the individual may seem simply a little scattered, a little shallow, and a bit self-centered. But as the disorder continues its path, the person with HPD exhibits far greater than the normal amounts of all these traits. As is the case with most personality disorders, HPD typically will decrease in intensity with age. Many who suffer from it will experience few of the most extreme symptoms by the time they are in their 40s or 50s.

Effects and Costs

HPD typically develops during adolescence and may have a negative effect on the person's capacity to function in social, occupational, or academic settings, resulting in failing to excel at school or maintain employment later in life (Kandola, 2017). Thus, left untreated, the disorder can cause problems in people's personal as well as professional lives.

Histrionic individuals are often described as overly theatrical. Unless they are the center of attention, they feel uncomfortable, disappointed—even angry—and may become flirtatious or provocative to achieve the desired attention. If their attempts fail, temper tantrums may follow in their disappointment.

Individuals with HPD may crave excitement, new things, and new experiences, which may lead to risky situations and eventually to increased depression. Another area of vulnerability for those afflicted with HPD is their suggestibility. In their exaggerated need for attention, they may gravitate toward a person they perceive to be important. When aligning themselves with such a person, histrionic individuals may readily follow that person's suggestions. This characteristic may also render them susceptible to scams by experienced "con men" (Dobbert, 2007).

Individuals with HPD tend to look for multiple people for attention within the social and romantic spheres. This may lead to marital problems due to jealousy and lack of trust from the other party, increasing the risk for divorce or separation (Disney, Weinstein, & Oltmanns, 2012). It may also affect their ability to cope with failures or losses and may lead to clinical depression. It is not uncommon for histrionic individuals, when unable to secure the desired attention, to become depressed, and they are actually at increased risk of suicide attempts.

In summary, histrionic individuals put themselves at risk of distress and disappointment when their theatrical attempts to gain the attention of those around them fail to bring the desired results. In desperation, they may step up their attempts to a more radical level, only to be shunned by those whose acknowledgment they seek. Finally, suicide attempts—often as theatrical as their other attention-seeking attempts—may follow in the expression of their disappointment. Usually, the suicide attempts are not valid attempts to kill themselves but a last effort to be acknowledged. Unfortunately for them, their ill-fated attempts at gaining attention result in more pain and disappointment. Furthermore, sometimes suicide occurs as result of unanticipated circumstances when all that was intended was a gesture.

In Society

People with HPD demand the role of "life of the party" with self-focused interests and conversation. They insist on being the center of attention in any group of people and may become uncomfortable, or even angry, when they are not receiving the desired acknowledgement. At other times, they may use their good social skills to manipulate others into acknowledging them and making them the center of attention (Cleveland Clinic, 2011). Generally, people with this disorder are able to function quite adequately in social settings, but at times they may embarrass their friends and acquaintances with public displays of affection or flattery, often embracing casual acquaintances with excessive ardor, or they may sob uncontrollably over minor sentimental situations. Their excessively impressionistic speech may at first captivate the attention of a listener, but the emotional style of their speech lacks congruity with the content, which is often lacking in detail. People observing those emotional displays may think that the histrionic individuals are faking these emotions because they are turned on and off so quickly. On the other hand, histrionic individuals are highly suggestible and easily influenced by others. They turn toward authority and powerful people, expecting their help while adopting their conventions and following their ideas, without necessarily following those ideas to the same depth as the authority figure.

People with an enviable social standing or fame constitute especially attractive targets to histrionic individuals, who hope to absorb some of the glamour for themselves just by being in the same room with them. In addition, at a later time, the situation can always be reported in the most glorious terms to the friends and acquaintances of the histrionic person. For people with this disorder, their self-esteem is dependent on the approval of others and does not grow from a true feeling of self-worth; therefore, it would seem logical for histrionics to associate with people of higher social standing because their approval would weigh in heavier on the self-esteem of the individual with HPD.

Often people with this disorder have strained or impaired relationships with same-sex friends because their sexually provocative interpersonal style may appear a threat to their friends' relationships. Furthermore, they may alienate friends with demands for constant attention (Bressert, 2016).

Histrionics become easily bored by routine activities. Their source of stimulation is in the novelty of experiences. Thus, long-term relationships are often neglected in favor of new friends. In the end, the histrionic individual often feels deserted; the new friends may become boring while previous stable friends have left the relationship due to the histrionic person's neglect of them (Bayer, 2000).

Up Close

All through his college years, Harlan had been the center of his group of friends. He participated in sports and took speech and acting classes along with his major in history. He hadn't decided whether he wanted to become a history professor or an actor. His father leaned strongly in the direction of history teacher. But Harlan was attractive and charming enough to make it as an actor, he thought. He dressed carefully so as to emphasize his attractive features. Perhaps his studies in history could qualify and enable him to play the roles of historically important men, Harlan thought. Although most of the time, he displayed a healthy self-confidence, inwardly he was not as strongly convinced of his abilities as he might have wanted to be. But the admiration of his friends helped, and that's why he tried so hard to get it. If he was not the center of whatever was going on, he worried, got bored, and became moody. There was nobody he could talk to at those times because he did not have any real close friends. Most of his social interactions occurred on a superficial level.

Harlan made sure he dated only the prettiest girls. It was important that his friends and classmates always envied him in addition to the admiration. His romantic relationships did not last long, because he was usually more interested in himself than in the young girl who was with him at the time. Women served a decorative purpose, just as his clothes did.

At Work

People with HPD may do relatively well in jobs that value and require imagination and creativity, but they will probably encounter difficulty with tasks that demand logical or analytical thinking. In addition, these individuals have a low tolerance for frustration and are easily bored by routine, often starting projects without finishing them or skipping from one event to another. As they crave novelty, stimulation, and excitement, they tend to become bored easily with their usual routine and frustrated by situations that involve delayed gratification. Frequent job changes may be the result.

Furthermore, histrionic people are lively, dramatic, vivacious, enthusiastic, and flirtatious. This combination can make the work place interesting and might even serve to increase productivity through enthusiasm; however, the flirtatiousness and overdramatic behaviors may also be disruptive to the work atmosphere and lead to rivalries among coworkers. In addition, the histrionic person's attention-seeking behavior may introduce an atmosphere of competition and even envy into the work situation, which may be disruptive in the overall work process.

Up Close

This morning Lynn spent more time than usual getting ready for work. She always dressed very carefully, making sure that the outfit chosen for the day made her blue eyes look even bluer and made her skin shimmer like pearls. Today was even more important because her boss had asked her to set time aside for a meeting. It would be a difficult meeting; Lynn had heard that there had been a work-related complaint about her. All the more reason to look as attractive as possible. It was almost an automatic reflex: whenever there were any problems, it was important that she look her best in an almost seductive way.

Lynn was intelligent and capable of performing her job as program manager, except that she got bored easily, and in trying to make work or her environment more exciting, she at times lost track of the individual parts along the complicated overall process of production. Lynn was not always aware when one of the workers in her team overlooked a step in the process or made a less-than-optimal decision. Usually, when the mistake was discovered, Lynn did not hesitate to blame the coworker for his or her forgetfulness or lack of expertise in handling the required details. Whatever the unfortunate situation turned out to be, it was never Lynn's fault. This was because she was usually thinking of the next project that might come her way. Newness made everything more exciting for Lynn.

The other part of Lynn's behavior that caused problems was her outrageous flirtatiousness. Every male employee and supervisor had experienced it. Some liked it—at least in the beginning—others were amused, and still others felt threatened, as if Lynn were trying to trick them into a dangerous situation where they might become victimized in some way. While Lynn joked and smiled flirtatiously, for some the work atmosphere around her became tense. And the other female employees did not like Lynn's seductive behavior toward the male employees, either.

It was no secret that Lynn had been divorced twice, and both times her husbands had complained about her being attracted to other men.

In Relationships

Histrionics' need to be at the center of attention in whatever event they are participating in may lead them to assign more significance than is actually justified to any relationship they are engaged in. Some of the people in those situations may be appalled by the exaggerated familiarity, while others may take advantage of the intimacy offered by the histrionic individual.

Mere acquaintances apparently become "best friends," as signaled by the histrionic person's behavior. Flirtatious or superficial romantic relationships may precipitate the delusion of deeply intimate associations in their minds, although in reality, they may have difficulty achieving true emotional intimacy in romantic relationships. They often act out a role, such as being a "princess" or a "victim" in their relationships with others. On one level, they may attempt to control their partner through emotional manipulation or seductiveness, while on another level, they may display a strong dependency on their partner (Bressert, 2016). Histrionic individuals' cognitive style is often superficial and lacking detail, which may not be conducive to the development of meaningful relationships.

Furthermore, while in a marriage or serious romantic relationship, the histrionic's flirtatious behaviors with others, possibly rivals (because those with HPD are more likely to look for multiple people for attention), may lead to divorce or dissolution of the relationship because the partner becomes tired of the apparent ongoing "competition" with the targets of the histrionic person's seductive behaviors. The histrionic person's self-centered attitude and lack of true concern for others may often leave partners of individuals with HPD with disappointment and the wish to exit the relationship.

Up Close

Melissa was facing her third divorce. Her marriages as well as her dating relationships were always of short duration. She was hungry for excitement, and being intimately involved with the same person became boring after a while, especially as Melissa had no real passion that gave her life meaning and that she could share with another person. Her verbal interchanges with others were lively but superficial and somewhat ambiguous, punctuated with smiles and expressive gestures.

Although she often acted seductively and wanted the man's sexual desire, she was not that interested in the physical part of sex. Always being attractive took work as well as some money; she didn't want all that to be disarranged by the groping hands of a man. Men usually misinterpreted her flirtatious and seductive behavior only to become disappointed after dating her for a while or being married to her. And Melissa could not allow them to stray and find with another woman what they had originally wanted from her—not while they were associated with her.

Melissa's life had become the perfect recipe for relationship breakups. The periods between relationships became longer and more frequent over time, and the depression that often filled those periods became stronger with every breakup. There had been a few suicide threats and even attempts over the years. Would this latest divorce be the trigger for another suicide attempt?

Theory and Research

A twin study conducted by the department of psychology at Oslo University explored possible correlations between genetics and Cluster B personality disorders. Using a test sample of 221 twins (92 monozygotic and 129 dizygotic twins), researchers interviewed the twins with the Structured Clinical Interview for *DSM-III-R* Personality Disorders (SCID-II). It was concluded that a correlation coefficient of 0.67 for HPD and genetic components indicated strong hereditary factors (Torgersen, 2000).

Another study, exploring "bright-side" Big Five Personality trait correlates of a "dark-side" personality disorder, namely hysterical personality disorder, included more than 5,000 British adult subjects completing the Neuroticism Extraversion Openness Personality Inventory Revised. The instrument measures the Big Five Personality factors at the Domain (Super Factor) and the Facet (Factor) level as well as the Hogan Development Survey (HDS), which includes a measure of HPD, exclusively called "Colourful" in the HDS terminology. Many of the associations between these "bright-" and "dark-" side individual difference variables were confirmed by correlation and regression results. The Colourful (HPD) score from the HDS was the criterion variable in all analyses. Colourful individuals are high on Extraversion and Openness but also on Stable and Disagreeable. The factor analysis identified Assertiveness and Immodesty as being particularly characteristic of that type. Previous work on HPD, using different population groups and different measures, was confirmed by this study, showing that personality traits are predictable and correlated with various personality disorders (Furnham, 2014).

Observations of a strong correlation between neurotransmitter function and Cluster B personality disorders such as HPD were reported in some studies. Individuals diagnosed with HPD seem to have highly responsive noradrenergic systems being responsible for the synthesis, storage, and release of the neurotransmitter norepinephrine. In general, high levels of norepinephrine lead to anxiety-proneness, dependence, and high sociability. Neurotransmitters communicate impulses from one nerve cell to another in the brain, and these impulses dictate behavior. The tendency toward an excessively emotional reaction to rejection—a trait that is common among HPD patients—may thus be attributed to a malfunction of catecholamines, a group of neurotransmitters (Lumen Learning, 2018).

A study regarding dependency needs in individuals diagnosed with HPD and DPD, using a Rorschach scale and a self-report inventory to measure dependency needs in HPD, found statistically significant correlation between HPD and high levels of tacit dependency needs. Women scored significantly higher than men on the interpersonal dependence inventory but seemed equal to men on the Rorschach scale, which also measured dependency needs. Self-report may also contribute to the higher diagnosis of HPD in women. There could be the expression of a strong cultural component in this as men are often socialized to mask such expressions of needs and emotions.

In addition, it was observed that dependency needs of the HPD individuals may be masked due to denial, displacement, and repression in a subconscious attempt to keep those needs out of their awareness (Bornstein, 1998).

Some researchers have expressed the opinion that many symptoms defining HPD in the DSM are exaggerations of traditional feminine behaviors. The findings from a peer and self-review study showed that femininity was correlated with histrionic, dependent, and narcissistic personality disorders (Klonsky et al., 2002).

There seems to be a strong gender bias among the psychological community relating to diagnosis in that women are much more frequently diagnosed with this disorder than men. Some studies have been conducted to explore such biases. In one study it was observed that in comparison to sex-unspecified vignettes, there was a high correlation with sex-specified vignettes and a tendency for clinicians to diagnose females as HPD and males with narcissistic personality disorder (Erickson, 2002).

For instance, when researchers randomly selected 354 psychologists and presented them with one of nine possible case histories, which reflected symptoms of HPD and ASPD, the clients in the case histories were described as male, female, or androgynous. The results showed a statistically significant gender bias within the diagnosis of personality disorders with a high tendency for female clients to be diagnosed as having HPD and for male clients to be diagnosed as ASPD (Ford & Widiger, 1989).

In another study, cited by Ford & Widiger (1989), 175 mental health professionals were presented with case histories consisting of mixed symptoms of both HPD and ASPD. It was found that female portrayed clients were diagnosed with HPD 76 percent of the time and ASPD 22 percent of the time. Male portrayed clients were diagnosed HPD 49 percent of the time and ASPD 41 percent of the time. The results reflected a tendency for therapists to perceive women as histrionic personalities and men as antisocial personalities—even when the patients exhibit identical symptoms.

The majority of observations regarding gender bias in personality disorders seems to indicate that when symptoms are identical, clinicians are more likely to diagnose HPD in women than in men and ASPD in men than in women (Garb, 1997; Morey, Alexander, & Boggs, 2005).

With the mention of histrionic personality disorder, there is usually a significant focus on its prevalent diagnosis in women compared to men as well as on its stereotypical criteria. This prompted a study, conducted by June Sprock (2000), published in the *Journal of Psychopathology and Behavioral Assessment*, involving a group of first- and second-year psychology students, who were separated into three different groups. The students were instructed to view the different criteria in the *DSM-III-R* and the *DSM-IV* and create three behavioral examples for the gender they were assigned or a neutral condition. The list was edited before it was sent to a group of psychiatrists and psychologists for their responses. Not surprisingly, feminine behaviors were rated more representative of HPD and somewhat more representative of the histrionic criteria than masculine behaviors, suggesting that the feminine sex role is more strongly associated with the label than the criteria. These results seem to provide a possible explanation for the higher rates of HPD in women.

Based on the notion of response modulation hypotheses of psychopathy, Cale and Lilienfeld (2002) explored the association between psychopathic, HPD, and ASPD features and performance on laboratory measures of passive avoidance errors and interference effects. Seventy-five theater actors were instructed to complete self-report questionnaires and two laboratory measures of response modulation, and peers completed questionnaires concerning the participants' personality disorder features.

The results showed only weak and inconsistent support for the hypotheses that HPD is a female-typed variant of psychopathy and that

ASPD is a male-typed variant of psychopathy. In contrast to previous observations, scores on response modulation tasks were not significantly related to psychopathy or to either HPD or ASPD.

In conjunction with the Epidemiological Catchment Area (ECA) survey conducted in Baltimore, Maryland, a two-stage probability sample of people in the community was developed with a full psychiatric examination using *DSM-III* criteria for HPD. The results reflected that this condition can be diagnosed reliably and that it is a valid construct with a prevalence of 2.1 percent in the general population, with males and females being equally affected. This would suggest that previous reports of an increased prevalence in women were expressions of ascertainment bias found in hospital-based studies. The diagnosis is associated with clear evidence of disturbance in the emotional, behavioral, and social areas. Individuals with this disorder appear to use health care facilities more frequently than do other people (Nestadt, Romanoski, Chahal, & Merchant, 2009).

A suggestion from one theory points toward a possible relationship between HPD and ASPD. Research found that two-thirds of patients who had been diagnosed with HPD also met criteria similar to those of ASPD (Barlow & Durand, 2005).

According to the *Encyclopedia of Mental Disorders*, HPD is seen mainly in men and women with above average physical appearances. It was suggested by some research that the connection between HPD and physical appearance holds for women but not necessarily for men. However, both women and men with HPD have a strong need to be the center of attention.

Also, HPD may be diagnosed more frequently in Hispanic and Latin American cultures and less frequently in Asian cultures, but more research is needed on the effects of culture upon the symptoms of HPD (Lumen Learning, 2018).

A study comparing a sample of women with HPD to an adequately matched sample of women without HPD (aged 24–31 years), using various measures, found women with HPD to have significantly lower sexual assertiveness, greater erotophobic attitudes toward sex, lower self-esteem, and greater marital dissatisfaction than the women without HPD. In addition, the women in the HPD group were found to experience significantly greater sexual preoccupation, lower sexual desire, more sexual boredom, greater orgasmic dysfunction, and a greater likelihood to enter into extramarital affairs than their counterparts. Despite these findings, the histrionic women reflected a higher sexual esteem. This pattern of sexual behavior noted among histrionic women seems to be consistent with behaviors exhibited in sexual narcissism (Apt & Hurlbert, 1994).

Concerned with the effectiveness of treatment with people with HPD, Kellett (2007) employed cognitive analytic therapy (CAT) in the treatment of a single case consisting of 24 CAT sessions and a 6-month follow-up period of four sessions. Data were collected to establish a baseline for HPD symptoms. Treatment outcome was judged according to the degree to which the key variables were reduced throughout the course of treatment. In addition, measurements were taken for positive changes that withstood the test of time after treatment. The following variables were measured daily: strong need to be noticed on a particular day, being focused on appearance on a particular day, being flirty on a particular day, feeling empty, and feeling like a child. The client's responses were measured on a scale from zero to nine. Furthermore, for reporting on those specified variables, the client was given a self-report measure of psychological functioning. This was administered at the onset of treatment, at termination, and again at the time of the final follow-up session.

The results of this case study presented statistically significant improvements in three of the five focal points for change. They were preoccupation with physical appearance, feelings of emptiness and feeling like a child inside.

At the onset of termination of the case study, problematic symptoms were exacerbated, most likely due to separation anxiety experienced by the patient, but over the long term and time withstanding, there was a reduction in problematic psychological functioning related to depression and personality integration.

Overall, there is no significant treatment research available for HPD. Two meta-analyses regarding psychotherapeutic treatments for personality disorders in general suggest that these conditions respond to both psychodynamic therapy and cognitive-behavioral therapy, but none of the included studies focused on HPD specifically. Most of the literature about this diagnostic entity has been written from a psychodynamic/psychoanalytic point of view. The lack of rigorously designed treatment trials on HPD leaves therapists to rely on accumulated clinical wisdom regarding the treatment of these patients.

Treatment

The recommended form of treatment for HPD is psychotherapy. Usually those who enter treatment do so because of symptoms of depression associated with dissolved romantic relationships rather than for an awareness of any histrionic symptoms related to the personality disorder. Therapy can be challenging because individuals with HPD may exaggerate their symptoms or ability to function. Also, they may be emotionally needy and challenge the boundaries set up by the therapist. Therapists' demonstration of empathy, understanding, appreciation, and willingness to listen may serve to reinforce the clients' symptoms of the disorder.

Unlike people who suffer from other personality disorders, those with HPD tend to seek treatment much quicker and exaggerate their symptoms and difficulty in functioning, although they seem to enter treatment at a more mature age, generally in their early 40s. In addition, because they are so emotionally needy, they are often reluctant to terminate treatment. Theoretical orientations most widely used in the treatment of HPD are psychodynamic and psychoanalytic approaches. Insight- and cognitive-oriented therapy approaches are considered by some to be ineffective in treatment of this disorder and should be avoided. The reasoning is that people with this disorder often are unable to examine realistically unconscious motivations and their own thoughts. As with BPD, because of the symptoms of their disorder, individuals with HPD may find themselves discriminated against by mental health professionals (Bressert, 2017).

In some experts' opinions group and family therapy approaches are generally not recommended for HPD clients because these individuals will often attempt to draw attention to themselves and exaggerate their actions and responses (Bressert, 2017).

Medication is not helpful in affecting the personality disorder, but medication may be used to help with the patient's depression that may follow disappointments. Treatment for HPD itself involves psychotherapy including cognitive therapy. Individual and group psychotherapy are likely choices to help patients recognize and confront their tendency to manipulate others and to find alternative ways to gain the reassurance they want.

Little research has been conducted regarding the actual effectiveness of treatment, leaving most emphasis on studying case histories (Kellett, 2007). Attempting to develop a treatment plan for HPD, a researcher divided it into three phases. The first stage consisted of stabilization, followed by the modification of communication techniques and style, and then finished with the modification of the client's interpersonal patterns, schemes, and reactions.

One of the most popular methods for assessing personality disorders is the unstructured self-inventory report. But with histrionic clients, there is the disadvantage of distortion in character, self-presentation, and self-image as rendered by the client. Most projective testing depends less on the ability or willingness of the individual to provide an accurate self-description, but there is only limited empirical evidence about the use of projective testing to assess HPD. Another preferred method is a semistructured interview, which tends to be more objective, systematic, replicable, and comprehensive (Sutker, 2002).

As a particular treatment approach for HPD, functional analytic psychotherapy is a way of identifying interpersonal problems with the patient as these problems occur, in session or out of session. The initial goals of functional analytic psychotherapy are determined by the therapist and include behaviors that fit the client's needs for improvement. The fact that the therapist directly addresses the patterns of behavior as they unfold in the session marks the difference between functional analytic psychotherapy and traditional psychotherapy.

Patients' in-session behaviors are considered to be examples of their patterns of poor interpersonal communication. The therapist must respond to the patients' behaviors and give feedback about how the behavior is affecting the therapeutic relationship during that time. In addition, the therapist assists clients with HPD by denoting behaviors that occur outside of treatment, the so-called "Outside Problems," hopefully leading to "Outside Improvements." In these sessions, a certain set of dialogue or script—called *coding client and therapist behavior*—can be utilized to provide clients with insight on their behaviors and reasoning (Callaghan, Summers, & Weidman, 2003).

The Functional Ideographic Assessment Template (FIAT) is another treatment example besides coding, used as a way to generalize the clinical processes of functional analytic psychotherapy. The template's purpose is to represent the behaviors that are a focus for this treatment. With it, therapists can create a common language to achieve stable and accurate communication results (Callaghan et al., 2003).

References

Alam, C. M., & Merskey, H. (1992). The development of hysterical personality. *History of Psychiatry, 3*(10), 135–165.

Apt, C., & Hurlbert, D. F. (1994). The sexual attitudes, behavior, and relationships of women with histrionic personality disorder. *Journal of Sex & Marital Therapy, 20*(2), 125–134.

Arthur, M. (2010). Histrionic personality disorder: Description, incidence, risk factors, causes, associated conditions, diagnosis, signs and symptoms and treatment. *Health.am*. Retrieved November 15, 2018, from http://www.health.am/psy/histrionic-personality-disorder/

Bakkevig, J. F., & Sigmund, K. (2010). Is the diagnostic and statistical manual of mental disorders, fourth edition, histrionic personality disorder category a valid construct? *Comprehensive Psychiatry, 51*(5), 462–470.

Barlow, D. H., & Durand, V. M. (2005). Personality disorders. In *Abnormal psychology: An integrative approach* (4th ed., pp. 443–444). Belmont, CA: Thomson Wadsworth.

Bayer, L. (2000). *Personality disorders.* Philadelphia, PA: Chelsea House Publishers.

Bienenfeld, D. (2007). Personality disorders. *Psychiatric Annals, 37*(2), posted February 1, 2007, healio.com.

Bornstein, R. (1998). Implicit and self-attributed dependency needs in dependent and histrionic personality disorders. *Journal of Personality Assessment, 71*(1), 1–14.

Bressert, S. (2016). Histrionic personality disorder symptoms. *Psych Central.* Retrieved August 2, 2017, from https://psychcentral.com /disorders/histrionic-personality-disorder-symptoms/

Bressert, S. (2017). Histrionic personality disorder treatment. *Psych Central.* Retrieved February 2, 2018, from https://psychcentral.com /disorders/histrionic-personality-disorder/treatment/

Cale, E. M., & Lilienfeld, S. O. (2002). Histrionic personality disorder and antisocial personality disorder: Sex-differentiated manifestations of psychopathy? *Journal of Personality Disorders, 16*(1), 52–72.

Callaghan, G. M., Summers, C. J., & Weidman, M. (2003). The treatment of histrionic and narcissistic personality disorder behaviors: A single-subject demonstration of clinical improvement using functional analytic psychotherapy. *Journal of Contemporary Psychotherapy, 33*(4), 321–339.

Cleveland Clinic. (2011). Histrionic personality disorder. Retrieved from http://www.clevelandclinic.org/health/health-info/docs/3700/3795 .asp?index=9743

Corbitt, E., & Widiger, T. (1995). Sex differences among the personality disorders: An exploration of the data. *Clinical Psychology: Science and Practice, 2*(3), 225–238.

Disney, K. L., Weinstein, Y., & Oltmanns, T. F. (2012). Personality disorder symptoms are differentially related to divorce frequency. *Journal of Family Psychology, 26*(6), 959–965.

Dobbert, D. L. (2007). *Understanding personality disorders: An introduction.* Westport, CT: Praeger Publishers.

Erickson, K. (2002). Psychologist gender and sex bias in diagnosing histrionic and narcissistic personality disorders. *Dissertation Abstracts International: Section B: The Sciences and Engineering, 62*(10-B), 4781.

Ford, M., & Widiger, T. (1989). Sex bias in the diagnosis of histrionic and antisocial personality disorders. *Journal of Consulting and Clinical Psychology, 57*(2), 301–305.

Furnham, A. (2014). A bright side, facet analysis of histrionic personality disorder: The relationship between the HDS Colourful factor and the NEO-PI-R facets in a large adult sample. *The Journal of Social Psychology, 154*(6), 527–536.

Garb, H. N. (1997). Race bias, social class bias and gender bias in clinical judgment. *Clinical Psychology: Science & Practice, 4*, 99–120.

Hales, E., & Yudofsky, J. A. (Eds.). (2003). *The American Psychiatric Press textbook of psychiatry*. Washington, D.C.: American Psychiatric Publishing.

Histrionic Personality Disorder. (1994). In *Diagnostic and statistical manual of mental disorders* DSM-IV (p. 667). Washington, D.C.: American Psychiatric Association.

Kandola, A. (2017). Histrionic personality disorder: Symptoms and diagnosis. *Medical News Today*. Retrieved February 4, 2018, from https://www.medicalnewstoday.com/articles/320485.php

Kaplan, M. (1983). A woman's view on DSM-III. (PDF). *American Psychologist, 38*(7), 786–792.

Kellett, S. (2007). A time series evaluation of the treatment of histrionic personality disorder with cognitive analytic therapy. *Psychology and Psychotherapy: Theory, Research and Practice, 80*, 389–405.

Klonsky, E. D., Jane, J. S., Turkheimer, E., & Oltmanns, T. F. (2002). Gender role and personality disorders. *Journal of Personality Disorders, 16*(5), 464–476.

Lumen Learning. (2018). Histrionic personality disorder. Retrieved June 21, 2018, from https://courses.lumenlearning.com/abnormalpsychology/chapter/histrionic-personality-disorder-2/

Millon, T. (2004). *Personality disorders in modern life*. Hoboken, NJ: John Wiley & Sons.

Morey, L. C., Alexander, G. M., & Boggs, C. (2005). Gender and personality disorder. In J. M. Oldham, A. E. Skodol, & D. S. Bender (Eds.), *Textbook of personality disorders* (pp. 541–554). Washington, D.C.: American Psychiatric Publishing.

Nestadt, G., Romanoski, A. J., Chahal, R., & Merchant, A. (2009). An epidemiological study of histrionic personality disorder. doi:10.1017/S003329100017724

Nolen-Hoeksema, S. (2014). Personality disorders. In *Abnormal Psychology* (6th ed., pp. 266–267). New York, NY: McGraw-Hill.

Pfohl, B., Personality disorder work group (1995). Histrionic personality disorder. In *Diagnostic and statistical manual of mental disorders, DSM IV* (pp. 655–658). Washington, D.C.: American Psychiatric Association.

Pinkofsky, H. B. (1997). Mnemonics for DSM-IV personality disorders. *Psychiatric Services, 48*(9), 1197–1198.

Psychology Today. (2018). Histrionic personality disorder. Retrieved March 6, 2018, from https://www.psychologytoday.com/us/conditions /histrionic-personality-disorder

Seligman, M. E. P. (1984). *Abnormal psychology.* New York, NY: W. W. Norton & Company.

Sprock, J. (2000). Gender-typed behavioral examples of histrionic personality disorder. *Journal of Psychopathology and Behavioral Assessment, 22*(2), 107–122.

Sutker, P. B. (2002). *Histrionic, narcissistic, and dependent personality disorders. Comprehensive handbook of psychopathology* (3rd ed., pp. 513–514). New York, NY: Kluwer Academic.

Tasca, C., Rapetti, M., Carta, M. G., & Fadda, B. (2012). Women and hysteria in the history of mental health. *Clinical Practice & Epidemiology in Mental Health, 8,* 110–119.

Torgersen, L., Olen, S., Onstad, E., Tambs, K., Svenn, S., Per Anders, I., . . . , Kristian, E. (2000). A twin study of personality disorders. *Comprehensive Psychiatric Journal, 41*(6), 416–425.

WebMD. (2018). Mental health and histrionic personality disorder. Symptoms, causes, treatments. Retrieved June 21, 2018, from https:// www.webmd.com/mental-health/histrionic-personality-disorder#1

CHAPTER 6

Narcissistic Personality Disorder

Symptoms, Diagnosis, and Incidence

The essential feature of narcissistic personality disorder (NPD) is considered to be a pervasive pattern of grandiosity, need for admiration, and a general lack of empathy for others and their discomfort. This pattern appears by early adulthood and is present in a variety of contexts.

In their grandiose sense of self-importance, individuals with NPD generally overestimate their own abilities and inflate their accomplishments to the point of being boastful and pretentious. In the inflated judgments of their own accomplishments and preoccupied with fantasies of unlimited success, power, and brilliance, they expect praise from others for their contributions and ruminate about "long overdue" admiration if the praise does not arrive.

Considering themselves to be unique, special, or superior, people with NPD may feel that only similarly unique or superior individuals can understand them and their special needs. Their insistence on only associating with equally special people may endow some of their acquaintances with elevated status just because they accept them conditionally, with the condition being eternal admiration.

The sense of entitlement in individuals afflicted with this disorder, combined with a lack of sensitivity to the needs of others, may result in their exploitation—conscious or not—of those around them. Although their self-esteem is usually fragile, their sense of entitlement seems designed to make up for it. The exaggerated focus on their own concerns may render individuals with NPD impatient and contemptuous with others who talk about their own problems, classifying those problems as signs of vulnerability or weakness. The often arrogant and haughty behaviors characteristic of people with narcissistic personality express the snobbish, disdainful, or patronizing attitudes they hold toward those around them.

Based on *DSM-IV* definitions, prevalence estimates for NPD range from 0 percent to 6.2 percent in community samples; about 50 percent to 75 percent of those diagnosed with narcissistic personality disorder are male. It has been suggested that the disorder's underreporting within criminal populations indicates a significantly higher percentage of males with the disorder than generally estimated (Dobbert, 2007).

It is believed that about 1 percent of all people are affected by the disorder at some point in their lives (Sederer, 2009). The previously observed higher frequency of NPD occurring in males than in females appears to be a continuing trend, and young people are affected more than older people (Caligor, Levy, & Yeomans, 2015). The disorder usually develops in adolescence or early adulthood, At times children or adolescents may exhibit some traits similar to those of NPD, but these traits may be transient and therefore do not meet the criteria for a diagnosis of the disorder (Mayo Clinic Staff, 2014).

In the World Health Organization's (WHO) *International Statistical Classification of Diseases and Related Health Problems 10th Revision ICD-10*, narcissistic personality disorder is listed under *Other specific personality disorder.*

Timeline

1898   British psychologist Havelock Ellis used the story of Narcissus to describe pathological self-absorption.

1914   Sigmund Freud offered a psychological discussion "On Narcissism."

1925   Robert Waelder first described the personality disorder.

1960s   Kohut and Kernberg suggested clinical strategies for using psychoanalytic psychotherapy with NPD patients.

1967   Kernberg introduced the term *narcissistic personality structure.*

1968   The current name came into use, proposed by Heinz Kohut.

History

The term "narcissism" to describe excessive vanity goes back to Narcissus, a mythological Greek youth who became infatuated with his own reflection in a lake. In popular culture, the condition of narcissistic personality disorder has been called megalomania (Parens, 2015).

Sigmund Freud commented on the neurotic's sense of omnipotence, regarding as a frank acknowledgment of the old megalomania of infancy, a megalomania that is essentially of an infantile nature and will be sacrificed to social considerations as development proceeds. Similarly, Edmund Bergler believed megalomania to be normal in the child; it may be reactivated later in life by gambling (Bergler, 1975). In Otto Fenichel's opinion, those individuals who react in later life with denial to narcissistic hurt, experience a regression to the megalomania of childhood (Fenichel, 1945).

As Freud regarded megalomania as an obstacle to psychoanalysis, in the second half of the 20th century object relations theory, officials both in the United States and among British Kleinians were reconsidering megalomania as a defense mechanism that might be potentially accessible for therapy. This approach would seem to be based on Heinz Kohut's view of narcissistic megalomania as an aspect of normal development, in contrast to Kernberg's consideration of such grandiosity as a pathological development distortion (Hughes, 2004).

NPD was first described by Robert Waelder, but the current name for the condition came into use in 1968 (O'Donohue, 2007). Reportedly, in December of 2010, it had been announced by the *New York Times* that the American Psychiatric Association might drop NPD as a recognized personality disorder in the next edition of the *Diagnostic and Statistical Manual of Mental Disorders* (DSM) (Goodman & Leff, 2012). However, whatever the considerations were at the time for possibly deleting the disorder, it is still represented in the *DSM-5*.

Narcissism has been considered by some to be a condition of the privileged. Theodore Millon and Roger Davis in their book *Personality Disorders in Modern Life* describe pathological narcissism as a condition of the royals and the wealthy (Goodman & Leff, 2012).

Theodore Millon suggested the following five subtypes of NPD: The *unprincipled narcissist* is characterized by pathological lying and deliberate deception in order to obtain narcissistic supply (the admiration of others). The *amorous narcissist* is obsessed with erotica and seduction. Sex and sex appeal are used as tools and weapons to gain control and power. The *compensatory narcissist* makes use of the narcissistic supply in order to compensate for overwhelming feelings of inadequacy and low self-esteem. The *elitist narcissist* shares the characteristics of the phallic narcissist, who is consumed with the external aspects of a superior manhood and is part of another classification system. But in contrast to the phallic narcissist, the class of elitist narcissists is not exclusively male (Goodman & Leff, 2012). And the *fanatic narcissists* are quite paranoid and believe that they are gods. Extreme delusions of grandeur are their weapons to fight their poor self-esteem. However, since there are few pure variants of any of the subtypes, they are not recognized in the *ICD* or *DSM* (Millon, 1996).

Another suggestion of subtypes of narcissistic personality disorder came from Will Titshaw, who identified the following three: *pure narcissists*, with mainly just NPD characteristics; *attention narcissists*, who also have histrionic features; and *beyond the rules narcissists*, who have antisocial features. These subtypes are also not officially recognized in any editions of the *DSM* or the *ICD*.

Development and Causes

The causes of NPD are not known, but experts suggest a biopsychosocial model of causation, indicating that a combination of environmental, social, genetic, and neurobiological factors is likely to play a role in the development. No single factor is responsible for the disorder; rather, it is thought that the complex and intertwined nature of all the considered factors is important. There is some evidence that NPD is heritable as it is more likely for individuals to develop it if there is a family history of the disorder, thus presenting a slightly increased risk for this disorder to be "passed down" to children (Paris, 2014).

Some authors believe that there is a relationship between NPD and the loss or absence of a strong father figure—that is, a father who is either physically or emotionally absent. Or the father may be condescending and critical, leaving the child with a lack of self-esteem, which the child later compensates for by exaggerating his or her own importance with a false sense of self-worth (Goodman & Leff, 2012).

Studies have indicated that narcissistic responses to stress and trauma may have a genetic basis, but there are additional factors at play. The potential for NPD may be in the genes, but environmental or other factors may be needed to set the disorder in motion. On the other hand, approximately two-thirds of the children of parents who were previously diagnosed with NPD have NPD themselves, according to some research (Goodman & Leff, 2012).

Researchers have established a list of factors that may promote the development of NPD. These include an oversensitive temperament; excessive admiration, praise, or criticism; overindulgences and overvaluation by parents or family members; severe emotional abuse; unpredictable or unreliable caregiving; learning manipulative behaviors from others; and valuing by parents in order to regulate the narcissistic individual's self-esteem (Groopman & Cooper, 2006). Cultural factors are also believed to influence the prevalence of NPD, as the traits seem to be more common in modern societies than in traditional ones (Paris, 2014).

Effects and Costs

Narcissists don't only lack empathy for others—they take advantage of others for their own ends. Such exploitative relationships may take many forms. They do not consider the losses or pain they inflict on others. Much of the emotional and material costs occur because NPD individuals can be very persuasive in getting what they want, and their victims often cannot believe that anyone could really be so cold and cruel.

As part of their strong beliefs in their own uniqueness and entitlement, many narcissists become addicted gamblers, expecting their friends and families to bail them out and cover their losses, even though the family members cannot afford to do so.

Narcissists' exaggerated need for attention and admiration may actually function as a risk factor for depression. At times, when the desired admiration fails to be available, the narcissist's disappointment may be as exaggerated as the original need for attention had been. Thus, depression becomes the price the narcissist often pays for the desired attention. In addition, narcissists' need for admiration can be interpreted as a dependency trait, and for many of them, drugs and alcohol may become a way to protect themselves from the harsh reality that they are not always the center of attention and admiration.

Drugs preferred by narcissists are those that stimulate their inflated sense of self and give them a feeling of euphoria and vitality and also fight feelings of disappointment and depression. One drug that provides all this is cocaine, and cocaine abuse is common among people with NPD (Goodman & Leff, 2012).

People who are in love with themselves tend to hate everyone else. For instance, in cases of racism and religious intolerance, narcissists are able to project all the qualities they despise onto the hated group, which leaves the narcissists with the "pure" selves they can love. The list of hated groups can include any religious sect, any race, minority, or nationality—except the ones the narcissists belong to (Grunberger, 1989).

As people with NPD have great difficulty tolerating criticism or defeat, they may be left feeling humiliated or empty upon experiencing an "injury" in the form of criticism or rejection (Psychology Today, 2017).

Narcissists' greatest vulnerability is a weak sense of self and the fear that others will see that. Theirs is a very thin, brittle facade of confidence and superiority. Once this thin veneer is punctured, narcissistic individuals may take things very personally, and they may hold onto resentments for a very long time. With only minor disappointments, narcissists may come up swinging, but when hit by a major blow to their self-concept, they may become totally deflated. They may even become suicidal (Hatch, 2017).

The greatest threat for people with NPD is the possibility of suicide because suicide attempts can arise quickly and without warning in those people (Links, Gould, & Ratnayake, 2003). The reason may be a sudden injury to the person's self-esteem.

In Society

As individuals with NPD are feeding their beliefs in their own importance and grandiosity from the admiration of those around them, they are only too eager to be socially involved—at least, on a superficial basis. Due to their lack of empathy, many of their social relationships remain on the superficial level.

NPD individuals' preoccupation with their own intelligence, success, and attractiveness tends to interfere with social interactions over longer periods of time because others do not appreciate, or tolerate for long, those competitive and admiration-demanding behaviors. In general, there seem to be two types of people with NPD: those who are outgoing in social situations and those who are not outgoing (Wink, 1991).

People with this disorder may frequently express their snobbish, disdainful, or patronizing attitudes when interacting with sales personnel in stores, food servers in restaurants, and many other public situations by complaining about the clumsy behavior, the rudeness, or stupidity of the people trying to complete their orders (Bressert, 2016).

Much like people with histrionic personality disorder, individuals with NPD crave attention from those around them, and they, too, may exaggerate the depth of their interpersonal relationships. But they are more likely to stress their friends' high social status. And persons with NPD are not just satisfied with attention, they expect to receive praise and admiration for their uniqueness and superiority (Bayer, 2000).

As they expect to be held in high esteem by others, they also believe that their specialness can only be truly understood and recognized by privileged people with social distinction. People with NPD firmly believe that they are entitled to special treatment. They expect to be seated at a special table in a restaurant, even though they did not bother making reservations. They will find something wrong with the meal and treat the server as second-class citizen, leaving a meager or no tip. The physicians they trust with their health issues have to be specialists in their field. They will attempt to join the most prestigious country club their income will allow. If they are not accepted into the prestigious country club, or they cannot afford to reside in the most affluent neighborhoods, they try to hide their failure by denigrating the neighborhood or the country club for being snobbish (Dobbert, 2007). While striving for the recognition of the social elite, narcissistic individuals will often behave in condescending or even offensive ways toward those who do not occupy the elevated social ranks.

The narcissists' sense of entitlement makes it easy for them to justify their exploitation of personal acquaintances and friends to their own advantage. Their assumed entitlement to the exploitation of those around them operates in every part of the narcissist's life.

It has been observed that narcissists tend to routinely use propaganda techniques to control, confuse, and manipulate others (Neuharth, 2017). The following is a list of some techniques used by narcissists:

Ad Hominem: From the Latin meaning "toward the man," this is an attempt to shift the conversation to questioning the other person's character or level of knowledge, thereby distracting from the topic and putting the other person on the defensive.

Glittering Generalities: Narcissists are in love with their words and use glowing statements describing themselves and their behaviors without providing evidence.

The Big Lie: Their lies are so outrageous that others don't even know where to begin in refuting them.

Intentional Vagueness: Being so vague in their statements so that they are meaningless or open to multiple interpretations.

Exaggerating and **Minimizing:** Most narcissists are extremely image conscious, so they minimize the negative parts of their actions and exaggerate when describing their grandiose personas.

Repetition: By endlessly repeating a word or phrase, narcissistic individuals sidetrack discussions. The goal is that if they say something often enough, others may finally start believing it.

Scapegoating: This is one of narcissists' favorite tactics: falsely blaming one person for a group's problems.

The basis for all these and other propaganda tactics is distortion of normal thinking and behavior for the purpose of misleading and exploiting others (Neuharth, 2017).

Up Close
Rita was the undisputed princess. Her parents, although not divorced, were separated, and her mother had taken in a foster child about two

years younger than Rita. The child payments from Rita's father, the money for Marion, the foster child, and additional money from the working mother of another neighborhood child, who was supervised by Marion, the foster child, allowed Mrs. Weimer to stay at home and raise both girls. Mr. Weimer drove a taxi for a living and did not spend much time with his estranged wife or with Rita.

Although Marion was the younger of the two girls, she was the one to help with all the chores around the house. Rita did not have to lift a finger. The neighborhood children liked Marion but would rather not play with Rita; she was too bossy and wanted everything to go her way. Whenever there was a fight among the children, Rita would tell her mother the story but switch her and Marion's roles in the children's upheaval; it was always Marion's fault. Marion could not defend herself because Rita threatened her that Mrs. Weimer would trade Marion for another foster child, a better one. Marion was too scared to risk another placement, which might even be worse for her, so she accepted Rita's power and suffered her abuse.

It did not help that Marion was a very pretty girl, much prettier than Rita. Rita could not allow that. She saw to it that Marion got to wear the ugliest hand-me-down clothing they could find. Sometimes, when Marion fell asleep, being exhausted from all the chores she had to do, Rita sneaked up and cut Marion's hair in the strangest pattern, telling her mother that Marion had done it herself to get attention. As Rita was not used to doing any work, her school performance was mediocre, and she barely graduated from high school. Mr. Weimer let it be known that child support for Rita would soon come to an end.

For a couple of years, Rita worked as a salesperson, but her personality traits were not conducive to that career. Rita expected to be treated as the star salesperson, making the most money and being admired by her less successful coworkers. Her unfriendly and haughty behavior with the customers, however, led to complaints, and she never lasted long in any of her jobs. But she never tired of blaming others for her failures. Finally she decided to become a bartender. It was easier to collect good tips by flirting with the male customers. And the bars she worked at usually did not have any other female bartenders, so the element of competition was not as obvious in this setting. She embarked upon a few ill-fated romantic relationships, with her disappointments leading to overeating and bouts with depression.

At Work

People with NPD are often charming and smart enough to do their jobs well in the beginning, but they soon get bored, and then they look for excitement. Changing their work routine may cause trouble, because they are not invested in the details and will try to blame coworkers for the problems. When a supervisor doesn't accept the blaming explanations, the person with NPD might sabotage coworkers' products, setting up traps for them and making it appear as if other coworkers set the traps, thus pitting one against another.

Narcissistic people do not do anything nice for others out of the kindness of their hearts—they don't have the empathy that that requires. Instead, they help out only to get more back in return. By getting positive feedback for gestures of seeming kindness, they verify that they are special.

Many people with NPD have the talent and credentials to function successfully in prestigious and powerful positions. Their pervasive social manner and charisma encourage casual business acquaintances. And they don't have to develop close relationships with anyone in the work situation. As pointed out by organizational psychologists, people with NPD are able to make necessary, tough business decisions without being bothered by emotions others would experience, such as sadness, empathy, or guilt.

Interestingly, a study about personality traits reported that politicians, clergy, and librarians scored highest on traits for authority and leadership, but they also had the highest scores in total narcissism values (Goodman & Leff, 2012).

Being part of a work group, the narcissistic worker proclaims the group's accomplishments to be his or her own achievements. Without his or her knowledge and skills, the group would have failed in its production.

Their sense of entitlement leads people with NPD to exploit colleagues in the work setting as they climb the corporate ladder. To meet their goals, narcissists don't mind stepping on others on the ladder to success. And if need be, they may not shy away from starting unfavorable rumors about those who are in competition with them (Dobbert, 2007).

Despite their self-perceived power and abilities, people with NPD are often lazy or feel above the need to show productivity in work activities. It is easier to fantasize about great achievements than to actually produce them in reality. They prefer their grandiose self-concepts in daydreams over realistic self-evaluations. This type of approach in the work setting will usually not reward the narcissistic individuals with the elevated and powerful positions they expect or demand to be functioning in. Therefore, in the workplace, narcissists often seethe with anger and resentment. Because the gap between their grandiose flights of fancy and reality is so great, they develop resentment, rage, and even persecutory delusions. In addition, they are extremely envious and try to destroy what they think to be the sources of their frustration, A successful boss, a popular coworker, a skilled employee—all become targets of the narcissist's competition and envy (Bjornlund, 2011).

Up Close

John, the older of two brothers, was intelligent, reasonably good looking, artistic, and had some charm. He made himself and everybody else, including his parents and his younger brother, believe that he was the one with the greatest potential. He only had a few friends, and they had to be willing to admire his brilliance and superior talents.

Although highly overrated by John, his intelligence allowed him to enter a promising career in the field of technology. He spent much time with his expensive technical toys and his musical instruments but expanded less energy on his work activities. However, he needed frequent raises in his salary to pay for the tools and toys he felt entitled to own. When his supervisor's performance ratings of John did not match John's own ratings, he blamed the supervisor for not being intelligent enough to recognize John's brilliance and superior performance. Sadly, the supervisor was just an ordinary man who somehow had made it up the ladder due to lucky circumstances or dishonest maneuvers.

According to John's beliefs, the supervisor, naturally, collected all the support he needed from John's coworkers, who envied him and talked about him behind his back.

As John had a tendency to express his dissatisfaction with his supervisor, frequent job changes were required. Strangely, all his supervisors seemed to come from the same mold. But, needing the money for his livelihood and his expensive toys, John was able to hold on to jobs, giving a less-than-stellar performance and using his energies for his hobbies and technical adventures.

Divorced after a disappointing marriage, John moved into a comfortable condominium with all his treasures. Unfortunately, his neighbors, to whom he seldom spoke because they were mostly just ordinary people, did not have any appreciation for the piano concerts he treated them to during late evening hours. How dare they demand he restrict his musical extravaganzas to the hours before 10:00 p.m.? They should have praised and thanked him for sharing his superior talents with them. Unfortunately for John, the law was on the side of his neighbors, the ordinary people.

Despite his difficulty interacting with supervisors, coworkers, neighbors, and others, John was able to keep some level of employment until he could retire with an adequate pension. At that time he left the con-dominium and moved into a small house out in the countryside, where he could indulge in his treasured activities without the distraction from friends, neighbors, and family. Not a bad life after all—in his opinion.

In Relationships

Due to the behavioral characteristics of people with NPD, it is often difficult to maintain romantic relationships (Campbell & Foster, 2002). Their inability to accept criticism of any kind and their demand for con-tinuing admiration and attention put a heavy burden on any intimate relationship. In addition, they may vent to their spouses their anger and disappointment over their colleagues' treatment of them at work and their supervisors' lack of understanding of the narcissist's grandiose achievements and contributions to the workplace, expecting their part-ners to soothe the wounds to their self-esteem and rebuild their exag-gerated self-confidence. However, when the spouse or partner is in need of emotional comforting, the narcissistic partner will rarely be avail-able because he or she might just be involved in another awe-inspiring project.

For people with NPD, any emotional interaction or any connection requiring an emotional commitment is doomed to failure. Surrounding themselves with people who will feed their narcissistic supply, they can-not express any real feelings of attachment or commitment and are thus unable to become part of a real friendship or love relationship. Partners of narcissistic individuals cannot afford to have or express their own opinions, because only the narcissists' opinions count; they alone have all the knowledge and are always right. And they will not forgive or forget any slight. Thus, relationships with narcissistic persons tend to be one-sided—physical, verbal, mental, financial, or emotional.

Within any type of relationship, four cycles of abuse—initiated and carried out by a narcissistic person—can be observed. As soon as the narcissistic person feels threatened, he or she embarks upon some sort of abusive behavior toward the person who appears to be responsible for the threat. Once the abuse cycle is in process, the individual with NPD will describe the victim's defensive behavior as evidence for that person's bad intentions, making him- or herself appear to be the victim. As soon as the real victim gives up in confusion, the narcissistic person feels empowered. Almost any perceived threat will trigger the abusive reactions within the narcissist, who will then turn the tables and assume the victim role that functions as justification to demonstrate his or her rightness or superiority, leading to increased power and control (Hammond, 2018).

The narcissists' strong belief in their own entitlement finds its expression in intimate relationships as well as in other parts of the narcissists' lives. Their willingness to share their lives with spouses or significant others entitles them to live in a smoothly functioning environment without their participation in making it so. It entitles them to sexual activity of their choosing at any time, and any concerns of a narcissistic person require immediate and undivided attention.

As many individuals with NPD are preoccupied with fantasies of unlimited success, brilliance, beauty, or even ideal love, their partners in close or intimate relationship most likely experience a rollercoaster of highs and lows in their daily lives with a narcissist. Consequences of unrealistic expectations of brilliance, power, and success in work situations will be aired at home, and more often than not, the partner's love for the narcissist does not match the level of ideal love fantasized or demanded by the narcissist.

Many narcissists tend to frequently behave seductively even to random people like compulsive seducers. They may believe that their worth is based on their looks, charm, and their ability to be sexually attractive to others (Hatch, 2017). Even if they are not actually cheating, this exaggerated seductiveness will introduce stress and problems into the narcissist's relationship with the intimate partner.

Narcissists have been described as living in a bubble surrounded by their own reflection (Goodman & Leff, 2012). There is no room for anybody else within the bubble.

Up Close

Because Martin believed that he was a special person, born to lead and guide the average people around him to a higher level, he also believed that he was the perfect lover. Secretly, some doubts sneaked in regarding his sexual performance after a few young women had broken up with him. To restore his beliefs in his special talents as a lover, he convinced himself that these pretty young women just did not recognize his stellar romantic performance. Then he decided to bestow his attention and amorous pursuits on some plain, overlooked young (and not-so-young) women. To give them a taste of the ecstasy of a perfect romance, he was on his most charming behavior for a while, lavishing his attention on them. He was generous with his sexual favors without wasting time inquiring what they might like. He knew he was entitled to their undying devotion in return. But when the women—after some initial happy excitement—returned to a lower level of excitement in the expression of

their sexual satisfaction, Martin was disappointed in the lack of grati-
tude expressed by them and decided to withdraw his generosity.

Theory and Research

The many similarities between narcissistic and paranoid personality disorders have made their distinction particularly difficult in some
researchers' opinions. Individuals with both types of disorders are ambitious, driven, haughty, and exhibit "narcissistic rage" when their pride
is injured. Developmentally, in both disorders, there are evidences of
an arrested separation-individuation, distorted Oedipus complex, and
a less-than-optimal latency and adolescent passage. On a psychostructural basis, subtle identity diffusion, often masked by an overzealous
but shallow vocational commitment, are noticeable in both disorders.
At some point it was even thought that cases with combined narcissistic and paranoid features may be more common than their pure types
(Akhtar, 1990). However, when this overlap is not strong, the two conditions show many differences. Individuals with NPD do not exhibit
the pervasive mistrust, litigiousness, and self-righteous indignation of
the paranoid personality. Narcissists tend to hide their discomfort with
spontaneity by crafty socialization, and cognitively, they display absent-
mindedness and lofty disregard for detail (Akhtar & Thomson, 1982).

According to studies on the occurrence of personality disorders in
twins, there seems to be a moderate to high degree of heritability for
NPD (Reichborn-Kjennerud, 2010). However, the specific genes and
gene interactions contributing to the cause have not been identified.

Based on the heritable traits and gender research, males with first-
degree biological relatives—most likely their fathers—diagnosed with
NPD have a higher likelihood of developing the same disorder (Dobbert, 2007). Suggestions from developmental psychologists indicate that
young people, especially young males, may develop NPD by observing
diagnosed narcissists modeling the symptomatic behaviors. In order to
understand the rewards or consequences associated with certain behaviors, it is not necessary to experience them directly. Individuals learn
behaviors by watching others perform the behaviors. If they like the consequences of the behavior, they are quite likely to imitate that behavior
and adopt it for their own use (Bandura, 1977).

Although there has been little research about the neurological basis
of NPD, recent research has identified a structural abnormality in
the brains of individuals with NPD. In particular, there seems to be a
smaller volume of gray matter in the left anterior insula (Schulze et al.,
2013). Similarly, another study has detected reduced gray matter in the

prefrontal cortex (Nenadic et al., 2015). The brain regions identified in those studies are related to the traits of empathy, compassion, emotional regulation, and cognitive functioning. These findings seem to indicate that NPD is linked to a compromised capacity for empathy and emotional regulation (Ronningstam, 2011).

A Norwegian study suggested that narcissism should be conceived as personality dimensions relevant to the whole range of personality disorders rather than as a distinct diagnostic category (Karterud, 2011). Another conclusion, based on examination of the literature on the disorder, suggested an apparent nosological inconsistency, indicating that its consideration as a trait domain needed further research (Alarcon & Sarabia, 2012).

A 2005 British study revealed significant elements of antisocial and narcissistic personality disorder among senior executives in the business sector (Bjornlund, 2011).

Theoretical considerations have focused on the split at the core of the narcissist's identity. Although people with NPD employ grandiose pretensions about themselves, their self-esteem is usually quite fragile, based on a secret self-image of helplessness and impotence. As a bulwark against this fragile self-image, which they fear is the more accurate picture, individuals with NPD have invented the "superman" representation of themselves. To compensate for this lesser self, which the narcissists secretly regard with shame, they invent their enormously inflated self-images. To make this attempted compensation more convincing even to themselves, narcissists have to manipulate other people into recognizing their grander selves (Bayer, 2000).

The defense mechanism of "splitting" in the narcissistic personality is considered to be similar to what is seen in the borderline personality. But there is a difference between the two types of splitting. The inner split in the borderline personality is more profound, and, unlike in the narcissistic personality, it brings with it alienation and rage (Restak, 1982).

For narcissistic individuals, feelings of inferiority and incompetence are among the most difficult to tolerate because of their shamefulness, and they are the most urgent to hide. Therefore, in order to protect the self from rejection, narcissistic individuals attempt to escape them by presenting a grandiose self and hiding the weaker self (Morrison, 1989).

Apparently, studies regarding the prevalence of NPD have found that rates of NPD are higher for young adults and for those individuals who were divorced, separated, or widowed than for the never married. In addition, significant cultural differences have been observed with black men and black and Hispanic women, reflecting higher rates of NPD in these groups than in Hispanic men and whites of both genders (Goodman & Leff, 2012).

Cultural trends in certain societal regions seem to contribute to the risk of developing NPD, according to social learning theorists. For instance, media centered on celebrities rather than on average people, importance placed on status and position, choice of leaders with emphasis on appearance and personality, and the weakening of religious and social institutions as part of traditional family life may lead to what has been called "acquired situational narcissism" affecting adults as a result of social successes, individuals who are always in the limelight, receiving special attention and recognition (Goodman & Leff, 2012).

This seems to be reflected by a study performed at the Keck School of Medicine, University of Southern California, which surveyed 200 celebrities using the Narcissistic Personality Inventory (NPI). As published in the *Journal of Research in Personality*, on average, celebrities scored 17.84 on the NPI, which is about 17 percent higher than the general public—with females scoring significantly higher than males. Of additional interest is that the research showed little or no relationship between the celebrities' NPI scores and the number of years they had been in show business. This finding was interpreted to mean that it is not show business and fame that led to narcissism, but rather that the individuals probably had narcissistic tendencies before they became famous (Goodman & Leff, 2012).

Recent theories have pointed to the influence of culture, socializations, lifestyle, pressures, and the media as influences that affect personality development in an overwhelming way—even as people grow into their 20s and beyond. And as pointed out by the Association for Body Image Disordered Eating (ABIDE), the average U.S. citizen is exposed to 5,000 advertising messages on a daily basis. Most of these messages are images of beautiful people with perfect bodies, enjoying the finer things in life. These messages are not only linked to eating disorders, they often provide a blueprint for the false images of perfection created by people with NPD.

People with NPD crave instant gratification, and digital technology seems to have been invented just for them. Cell phones provide the means to create a self-centered environment for oneself by only interacting with those peers whom one can rely on to feed one's narcissistic tendencies. The various social network sites can be easily manipulated for building a network of fans and followers by screening out those individuals who hold different opinions from those of the narcissist. On those social networking sites, the narcissist can be the center of his or her world, reflecting it nonstop to the circle of admirers. Narcissists are susceptible to developing Internet addiction. In a recent study, two-thirds of young participants stated that as a whole, their generation was more overconfident, more narcissistic, and more needy for instant gratification and attention than those of their parents' and earlier generations (Goodman & Leff, 2012).

There has been some controversy questioning the actual existence of a distinct emotional disorder to be called "narcissism" or NPD, and there was a suggestion to remove NPD from the diagnostic literature as a separate personality disorder because many psychological disorders have a degree of narcissism in them. This led to confusion about NPD being the same as or being a type of schizophrenia. A study designed to show that NPD was a separate condition from schizophrenia involved a group of patients hospitalized and treated for a diagnosis of NPD, comparing them to a group of patients hospitalized for schizophrenia in terms of therapy effectiveness and clinical outcomes. The conclusion, based on the results, was that NPD constitutes a valid diagnostic entity, distinct from schizophrenia (Goodman & Leff, 2012).

Many people seem to believe that there is a narcissistic epidemic in the United States, starting with the so-called "me decade" of the 1970s, when admiring oneself came to be equated with success in life. This idea turned into something like a movement in the 1980s and 1990s, becoming the age of entitlement. Using statistics, some point out that based on changes in averages, narcissism has reached an epidemic. The level of change in narcissistic traits in today's population—as opposed to the early 2000s—represents a classic bell curve, with small changes at the middle (the average) and much greater changes at the ends. Looking at the top of the bell, the average person is only somewhat narcissistic, although noticeably more so now than a decade ago. However, at the high end of the bell curve, there are now three to four times as many people diagnosed with NPD than there were a decade ago, indicating that there are many more highly narcissistic people with us now than one or two decades ago (Goodman & Leff, 2012).

According to some research, NPD tends to be exhibited more often in people with higher education and in certain professions. For instance, a study of personality traits published in the journal *Current Psychology* noted that the highest scores on traits for leadership and authority, but also the highest scores in total narcissism values, were obtained by politicians, clergy, and librarians.

Treatment

Historically speaking, for many years it was believed that it was nearly impossible to treat people with NPD, but although it is very difficult to convince someone with NPD to change his or her behavior, it is not impossible (Goodman & Leff, 2012).

In the 1960s, the conventional wisdom of the time was challenged by Heinz Kohut and Otto Kernberg, who outlined clinical procedures for using psychoanalytic psychotherapy with clients with NPD that they claimed were effective in treating the disorder. Contemporary treatment modalities typically involve transference-focused, metacognitive, and schema-focused therapies. Treatment of symptoms related to comorbid disorders with psychopharmaceuticals might provide some improvement. But, according to Elsa Ronningstam from Harvard Medical School, "alliance building and engaging the patient's sense of agency and reflective ability are essential for change in pathological narcissism" (Ronningstam, 2016, p. 11).

Treatments of NPD have not been well studied, and many people afflicted with the condition frequently do not consider themselves to have a problem. If they do enter treatment, it may be for another complaint, such as depression or substance use disorder—or at the insistence of relatives. Because of their extremely positive self-image, they fail to recognize their behavior as inappropriate (Caligor, Levy, & Yeomans, 2015). They resist the notion that they could be damaged in any way. Thus, because people with NPD exhibit grandiosity and defensiveness, treatment can be challenging. However, individual and group psychotherapy may be useful in helping them relate to others in a healthier and more compassionate way.

Several therapy approaches have been suggested as effective ways of treating NPD, including mentalization-based, transference-focused, and schema-focused psychotherapies (Psychology Today, 2017). Heinz Kohut and Otto Kernberg in the 1960s claimed their clinical strategies for using psychoanalytic psychotherapy with NPD clients. Contemporary treatment approaches involve transference-focused, metacognitive, and schema-focused therapies.

Medications may be prescribed to relieve specific troubling and debilitating symptoms. Some of the SSRI (selective serotonin reuptake inhibitors) class of antidepressants, such as Prozac, may actually tend to increase narcissistic traits. As the neurotransmitter serotonin regulates mood and levels of positive emotions, stimulating normal positive emotions, it may at the same time also stimulate the false feelings of superiority typical of people with NPD (Goodman & Leff, 2012).

Psychopharmaceuticals may be useful in the relief of symptoms related to comorbid disorders, but alliance-building and engaging the patient's sense of agency and reflective ability are necessary for change to occur (Ronningstam, 2016). As mentioned earlier, people with NPD do not acknowledge having problems, instead believing that everybody else is to blame for whatever problems arise. If—for whatever reason—they enter therapy, their attitude makes psychotherapy difficult because they fear that making changes in themselves would represent an admission of their imperfection.

One published account of therapy describes a male patient who admitted that he had never really loved anyone, even though he had been in a number of romantic relationships. Apparently, he felt some guilt over having for years let others love him without reciprocating the feeling. But whenever this topic came up in therapy, the client would fall asleep in order to hide from his shame (Bach, 1985).

However, in spite of these difficulties, psychotherapy seems to be the preferred method for dealing with narcissism. In fact, family or group therapy can at times be helpful because the narcissist's difficulties dealing with other people become evident immediately in such settings, although ultimately, individual psychotherapy may be necessary for uncovering dramatic childhood events that might have prompted the development of the individual's elaborate defense system (Bayer, 2000).

References

Akhtar, S. (1990). Paranoid personality disorder: A synthesis of developmental, dynamic, and descriptive features. *American Journal of Psychotherapy, 44*(1), 5–25.

Akhtar, S., & Thomson, A. J. (1982). Overview: Narcissistic personality disorder. *American Journal of Psychiatry, 139*, 12–20.

Alarcon, R. D., & Sarabia, S. (2012). Debates on the narcissistic conundrum: Trait, domain, dimension, type, or disorder? *Journal of Nervous and Mental Disorders, 200*, 16–25.

Bach, S. (1985). *Narcissistic states and the therapeutic process.* New York, NY: Jason Aronson.

Bandura, A. (1977). *Social learning theory.* Englewood Cliffs, NJ: Prentice Hall.

Bayer, L. (2000). *Personality disorders.* Philadelphia, PA: Chelsea House Publishers.

Bergler, E. (1975). The psychology of gambling. In J. Halliday & P. Fuller (Eds.), *The psychology of gambling* (pp. 176–182). London: HarperCollins Publishers.

Bjornlund, L. (2011). *Personality disorders.* San Diego, CA: Reference Point Press.

Bressert, S. (2016). Narcissistic personality disorder: Symptoms & treatment. *Psych Central*. Retrieved July 31, 2017, from https://psychcentral .com/disorders/narcissistic-personality-disorder-symptoms/

Caligor, E., Levy, K. N., & Yeomans, F. E. (2015). Narcissistic personality disorder: Diagnostic and clinical challenges. *The American Journal of Psychiatry, 172*(5), 415–422.

Campbell, W. K., & Foster, C. A. (2002). Narcissism and commitment in romantic relationships: An investment model analysis. *Personality and Social Psychology Bulletin, 28*, 484–495.

Dobbert, D. L. (2007). *Understanding personality disorders: An introduction.* Westport, CT: Praeger Publishers.

Fenichel, O. (1945). *The psychoanalytic theory of neuroses.* New York, NY: Norton.

Goodman, C. L., & Leff, B. (2012). *The everything guide to narcissistic personality disorder.* Avon, MA: Adams Media.

Groopman, L. C., & Cooper, A. M. (2006). Narcissistic personality disorder. *Personality Disorders—Narcissistic Personality Disorder.* Armenian Health Network 2 July 2, 2010, health.am.

Grunberger, B. (1989). *New essays on narcissism.* London: Free Association Books.

Hammond, C. (2018). The narcissistic cycle of abuse among siblings/ The exhausted woman. *Psych Central. Professional.* Retrieved April 03, 2018, from propsychcentral.com

Hatch, L. (2017). Are you a narcissist? *Psych Central.* Retrieved October 25, 2017, from https://blogs.psychcentral.com/sex-addiction/2017/10 /are-you-a-narcissist/

Hughes, J. M. (2004). *From obstacle to ally: The evolution of psychoanalytic practice.* London: Routledge.

Karterud, S. (2011). Validity aspects of the Diagnostic and Statistical Manual of Mental Disorders, Fourth Edition, narcissistic personality disorder construct. *Comprehensive Psychiatry, 52*(5), 517–526.

Links, P. S., Gould, B., & Ratnayake, R. (2003). Assessing suicidal youth with antisocial, borderline, or narcissistic personality disorder. *Canadian Journal of Psychiatry, 48*(5), 301–310.

Mayo Clinic Staff. (2014). Narcissistic personality disorder: Symptoms. *Mayo Clinic.* Retrieved April 29, 2016, from http://www .mayoclinic.org/diseases-conditions/narcissistic-personality-disorder /con-20025568

Millon, T. (1996). *Disorders of personality: DSM-IV-TM and beyond* (p. 393). New York, NY: John Wiley and Sons.

Morrison, A. P. (1989). *Shame: The underside of narcissism.* Hillsdale, NJ: Analytic Press.

Nenadic, I., Güllmar, D., Dietzek, M., Langbein, K., Steinke, J., & Gader, C. (2015). Brain structure in narcissistic personality disorder: A VBM and DTI pilot study. *Psychiatry Research, 231*(2), 184–186.

Neuharth, D. (2017). 12 Classic propaganda techniques narcissists use to manipulate you. *Psych Central.* Retrieved September 13, 2017, from https://blogs.psychcentral.com/narcissism-decoded/2017/09/12 -classic-propaganda-techniques-narcissists-use-to-manipulate-you

O'Donohue, W. (2007). *Personality disorders: Toward the DSM-V* (p. 235). Los Angeles, CA: SAGE Publications. Retrieved from https:// books.google.com/books?id=A7ODnQJnD74C&pg=PA235

Parens, H. (2015). *War is not inevitable: On the psychology of war and aggression* (p. 63). Lanham, MD: Lexington Books.

Paris, J. (2014). Modernity and narcissistic personality disorder. *Personality Disorders: Theory, Research, and Treatment, 5*(2), 220.

Psychology Today. (2017). Narcissistic personality disorder. Retrieved August 2, 2017, from https://www.psychologytoday.com/conditions /narcissistic-personality-disorder

Reichborn-Kjennerud, T. (2010). The genetic epidemiology of personality disorders. *Dialogues in Clinical Neuroscience, 12*(1), 103–114.

Restak, R. M. (1982). *The self-seekers.* New York, NY: Doubleday.

Ronningstam, E. (2011). Narcissistic personality disorder: A clinical perspective. *Journal of Psychiatric Practice, 17*(2), 89–99.

Ronningstam, E. (2016). New insights into narcissistic personality disorder. *Psychiatric Times, 33*(2), 11.

Schulze, L., Dziobek, I., Vater, A., Heekeren, H. R., Bajbouj, M., Renneberg, B., . . . Roepke, S. (2013). Gray matter abnormalities in patients with narcissistic personality disorder. *Journal of Psychiatric Research, 47*(10), 1363–1369.

Sederer, L. (2009). *Blueprints psychiatry* (5th ed., p. 29). Philadelphia, PA: Wolters Kluwer/Lippincott Williams & Wilkins. Retrieved from https://books.google.com/books?id=7_7-5dQlpBQC&pg=PA28

Wink, P. (1991). Two faces of narcissism. *Journal of Personality and Social Psychology, 61*(4), 590–597.

CHAPTER 7

Obsessive-Compulsive Personality Disorder

Symptoms, Diagnosis, and Incidence

As the name implies, people who suffer from obsessive-compulsive personality disorder (OCPD) are plagued with thoughts or ideas that stay in their minds and are difficult to dismiss. On the other hand, compulsion refers to a type of behavior that the individual feels driven to perform. This personality disorder should not be confused with the more serious anxiety condition called *obsessive-compulsive disorder* (OCD). Strictly speaking, individuals with OCPD do not have any one identifiable obsession or compulsion but rather tend to be utter perfectionists, insisting that everything must be done in certain ways. They are unlikely to compromise (Bayer, 2000).

Although unusual, it is possible for an individual to suffer from both disorders, particularly in extreme cases of hoarding behavior. For instance, in cases of animal hoarding, it has been reported that the people involved appear to have symptoms of both OCD and OCPD (mind-disorders.com, 2018).

A preoccupation with orderliness, perfectionism, and interpersonal control at the expense of flexibility and efficiency make up the essential feature of OCPD, which usually starts in early adulthood. Painstaking attention to rules, trivial details, schedules, and procedures are among the tools people with OCPD employ in attempting to remain in control. Their repeated checking for possible errors may become annoying to those around them due to delays and inconveniences resulting from this behavior.

People with OCPD are high achievers with a sense of urgency about their actions. If other people interfere with their rigid routines, they may become very upset and may not be able to express their anger directly because they consider feelings like anxiety or frustration more appropriate than anger. Rather than expressing their angry feelings, they may ruminate for hours about the situation, thereby increasing the level of their frustration.

Individuals with OCPD usually exhibit excessive devotion to work—often to the exclusion of leisure activities and interaction with friends—which is not necessarily dictated by economic necessity. Even on vacations, they may take along something to work on to avoid "wasting time." Play becomes a structured task, and hobbies are approached as serious tasks that demand careful planning and organization to be mastered perfectly. In addition, people with OCPD are reluctant to delegate tasks or work together with others.

Regarding matters of morality, ethics, or values, individuals with OCPD are inflexible and conscientious, forcing themselves and others to uphold rigid moral principles and the strictest standards of performance. They defer to authority and rules, insisting on literal compliance without regard for extenuating circumstances.

People with this disorder tend to be stingy and hoard money. They also have great difficulties discarding objects that are no longer needed because there could be a time in the future when they could be useful again. And they may adopt a standard of living that is far below their actual financial means. As rigidity and stubbornness are main characteristics of OCPD, people with this disorder have difficulty compromising with the ideas of others because there is only one "correct" way for things to be done. It is problematic for them to acknowledge the viewpoint of others, and they are unwilling to consider changes in their opinions as well as their behavior.

OCPD is one of the most frequently occurring personality disorders in the general population with an estimated prevalence range of 2.1 percent to 7.9 percent and 8 percent to 9 percent among psychiatric outpatients. Other estimates suggest that approximately 1 percent of the general population is affected by the disorder (Bayer, 2000). Results of systemic studies indicate that OCPD tends to be diagnosed about twice as often in males than in females. Some research appears to link this disproportion to gender stereotyping in that men have greater permission from general Western culture to act in stubborn, withholding, and controlling ways. The cultural permission, while encouraging men to behave in controlling ways, may also serve to "camouflage" this condition in men. In other words, the prevalence rate of OCPD in men may even be higher than estimates reflect.

Starting in the teen years or early 20s, OCPD is currently the most prevalent neurotic character structure, partly because the disorder makes it possible for people to achieve the illusion of safety in an uncertain world (Salzman, 1968). A large U.S. study reported a prevalence rate of 7.9 percent, making OCPD the most common personality disorder. The data evaluation regarding the prevalence, sociodemographic correlates, and disability of 7 of the 10 *DSM-IV* personality disorders revealed OCPD to be the most prevalent personality disorder in the general public (contradicting other information), with no sex differences being observed. Regarding its role in prediction of disability, OCPD was inconsistently related to disability (Grant et al., 2004).

Some traits of OCPD may seem to occur in other personality disorders; for example, a person with narcissistic personality disorder may be preoccupied with perfection and show a stingy and critical attitude toward others. In general, narcissists are generous with themselves, but people with OCPD are self-critical and reluctant to spend money even on themselves. Similarly, individuals with schizoid personality disorder, who lack a fundamental capacity for intimacy, may resemble someone with OCPD in being very formal and detached in interactions with others. What is different is that a person with OCPD may be awkward in emotional situations but is still able to experience caring and may actually long for close relationships.

Timeline

1908   Sigmund Freud named what is now known as obsessive-compulsive personality disorder "anal retention character."

History

OCPD has a lengthy history, tracing back to the beginnings of psychology. It has appeared in every edition of the *DSM*. Sigmund Freud identified the main characteristics of the personality type as a preoccupation with orderliness, parsimony (frugality), and obstinacy (stubbornness and rigidity). The concept agrees with his theory of psychosexual development.

When OCPD was first included in *DSM-II*, it was largely based on Freud's notion of the obsessive personality or anal-erotic character style exemplified by orderliness, parsimony, and obstinacy.

OCPD's *Anankastikos* diagnostic criteria (the World Health Organization's ICD-10 uses the term *anankastic personality disorder*; derived from the Greek word *Anankastikos*: "compulsion") have undergone considerable changes with each DSM modification. For example, two criteria listed in the *DSM-III-R*, constrained expression of affection and indecisiveness, were discontinued in the *DSM-IV*. This occurred mainly as a result of reviews of the empirical literature, which found that these traits did not contain internal consistency. Research regarding characteristics of OCPD and its core features has been ongoing since the early 1990s, including the tendency for it to run in families, along with eating disorders.

In the *DSM-IV*, OCPD is classified as a Cluster C personality disorder although there had been a dispute about OCPD's categorization as an Axis II anxiety disorder. It seemed more appropriate for OCPD to be presented alongside OC spectrum disorders including OCD, compulsive hoarding, body dysmorphic disorder, trichotillomania, compulsive skin picking, tic disorders, autistic disorders, and eating disorders (Fineberg, Sharma, Sivakumaran, Sahakian, & Chamberlain, 2007).

There has been a note of criticism regarding the inclusion of OCPD as a Cluster C disorder. The findings of a 2007 study indicated that OCPD is etiologically distinct from avoidant and dependent personality disorders, thereby suggesting that OCPD is incorrectly categorized as a Cluster C disorder (Reichborn-Kjennerud et al., 2007).

The *DSM-IV* tried to distinguish between OCPD and OCD by focusing on the absence of obsessive and compulsive traits in OCPD, but OC personality traits are easily mistaken for abnormal cognitions considered to be basic to OCD. Parts of self-directed perfectionism, such as believing a perfect solution is commendable, discomfort if things are believed to have been done incompletely, and questioning whether one's actions were performed correctly, have also been suggested as enduring features of OCD. And in *DSM-IV* field trials, a majority of OCD patients stated they were unsure whether their obsessive-compulsive symptoms really were unreasonable (Foa et al., 1995).

In 2004, Theodore Millon identified the following five subtypes of the compulsive personality: perfectionism, inflexibility, rule-bound, doubt and cautiousness, and order and symmetry; any compulsive personality may exhibit one or more of them (Millon, 2004).

Development and Causes

Individuals with OCPD are thought to have not experienced a successful separation-individuation process and to have not acquired self- and object-constancy. According to the psychoanalytical view, their problem seems to develop from oedipal-phase difficulties.

Others suggest that the need for control may stem from traumatic losses early in life, such as the death of a parent. The powerlessness in averting this past tragedy may drive those with an obsessive-compulsive personality to rule or control as much as possible within their present reality (Bayer, 2000).

Several theories suggest that people with OCPD may have been raised by controlling or overprotective parents. Or, as children, they may have been harshly punished and may have developed OCPD traits as a coping mechanism to avoid punishment by trying to be obedient and "perfect" (Van Noppen, 2010).

According to some research, people with OCPD appear to have been raised by parents who punished them for every transgression of a rule, no matter how minor, and rewarded them for almost nothing. This treatment leaves children unable to safely develop or express a sense of joy, spontaneity, or independent thought, and they develop the symptoms of OCPD as a strategy for avoiding punishment. This type of upbringing may lead children to suppress the anger they feel toward their parents. Acting outwardly in an obedient manner, they may be polite toward authority figures, but at the same time, they may treat younger children or those they regard as their inferiors harshly. So far, genetic contributions to OCPD have not been well documented. It is possible, however, that cultural influences may play a part in the development of OCPD. Highly authoritarian and rule-bound cultures may encourage child-rearing practices that contribute to the development of OCPD. Similarly, some religions and professions require exactness as well as careful attention to rules in their members. However, there is reason for caution: as such information is becoming easily accessible to the general public, it is not surprising to see some parents of individuals with OCPD taking extreme offense to it (Mind Disorders, 2018).

The exact cause of OCPD is not known, but there are several theories about the possible causes. Most professionals subscribe to a biopsychosocial model of causation, with no single factor having the sole responsibility. Instead, it seems that it is the complex and likely intertwined nature of all three factors that is important. There are also indications that there is a slightly increased risk for this disorder to be "passed down" to the next generation (Bressert, 2017).

OCPD is a distinct disorder from OCD, and the relationship between the two disorders is contentious. Some studies report high comorbidity rates between the two disorders. They may also share outside similarities, such as rigid and ritual-like behaviors. Furthermore, orderliness, hoarding, and a need for symmetry and organization are often found in people with either disorder. But the attitudes toward these behaviors differ between people afflicted with either of the behaviors. People with OCD do not want these behaviors and regard them as unhealthy, as the product of anxiety-inducing and involuntary thoughts. For people with OCPD, on the other hand, these behaviors are egosyntonic (perceived by the subject as rational and desirable), like being the result of a strong adherence to routines, natural inclination toward cautiousness, or a wish to achieve perfection.

Persons affected by OCPD often find it difficult to relax, always fearing that time is running out for their activities and feeling that more effort is needed to achieve their goals. Their planning of activities down to the minute is a manifestation of the compulsive tendency to keep control over their environment and their dislike of unpredictable events that they cannot control.

Effects and Costs

Some OCPD patients have an obsessive need for cleanliness, often combined with an obsessive preoccupation for tidiness. This obsessive tendency could make their daily lives quite difficult. Even though this type of obsessive behavior can bring about a sense of "controlling personal anxiety," tension might continue to exist. On the other hand, people with OCPD might tend to not organize things; they might become compulsive hoarders, and they could be hindered by the amount of clutter that they still plan to organize at some point in the future. In reality, OCPD patients might not ever do obsessive cleaning and organizing as they become busier with their workload, which might turn their stress to anxiety (Jefferys & Moore, 2008).

OCPD's main symptoms of preoccupation with remembering past events, attending to minor detail, excessive compliance with existing social customs and rules, unwarranted compulsion to note-taking or list-making, and rigidly holding on to beliefs or showing unreasonable degrees of perfectionism could eventually interfere with completing the task at hand.

The symptoms of OCPD may cause different levels of distress for varying periods of time (transient, acute, or chronic), interfering with the person's occupational, social, and romantic life. The social isolation and difficulty with handling anger that are common in people with OCPD may lead to depression and anxiety later in life. People with OCPD frequently lean toward general pessimism or depression, which, at times, can become so serious that suicide becomes a risk (Pinto, 2014).

A distinctive aspect of OCPD, in comparison with most mental disorders, is its inconsistent relationship with psychosocial functioning. While OCPD can interfere significantly with social and romantic relationships, it has also been shown to relate positively with educational attainment, career success, and wealth (Samuel & Griffin, 2015).

In Society

People with OCPD regard their moral dictates to be unquestionably superior to their instinctual desires and to the moral dictates of most other people. They believe that others should behave as they do. When others don't follow the rules, or if they have to wait in line for something, people with this disorder get upset or angry. But they usually don't express their anger in constructive ways; instead, they tend to ruminate about the reason for the anger. Generally, emotions are expressed by individuals with OCPD in a stylized, stilted fashion.

In situations without clearly defined rules, those with OCPD are often anxious because they are afraid that they might make a mistake and get punished for it. People afflicted with this disorder may have difficulty learning a new route to a familiar place.

An additional characteristic of this personality disorder is stinginess or miserliness, often combined with an inability to throw away worn-out or useless items, leading to the person suffering from "pack rat" behavior.

People diagnosed with OCPD often come across to others as difficult and demanding. Interestingly, their rigid expectations of others are also applied to themselves, as they are just as intolerant of their own shortcomings. They feel forced to present a consistent facade of propriety and control.

Up Close
Nancy, the scheduling manager in the service department of a local automobile dealership, was extremely efficient and extremely slim. One of

the many perfectionist aspects of her life involved a rigid eating ritual. At the end of a meal, her plate was never empty; there was always at least one bite of food left. Nancy praised herself for every food item she did not put into her mouth. In fact, the leftover food items were more gratifying to her than the food she ate. Eating all the items on her plate would make her fear that she might go for a second helping and eventually lose control to the point where she could not stop eating ever again.

Observing Nancy's mealtime behavior, most people thought it was her way of keeping herself on a strict diet. Nancy's slim figure seemed to be a confirmation of that notion, but that was only part of the reason. Actually, Nancy's rigid eating behavior was in response to her mother's controlling behavior, when she made Nancy eat all the food on her plate whether she was hungry or not. No excuse to leave some food on her plate was accepted by her mother, who often made Nancy sit alone at the dinner table for hours until the last morsel was gone. At first, Nancy had tried to hide some of the unwanted food items under the rug, but her mother detected the food and made her eat it right then and there, with some hairs or threads from the rug sticking to the food. The punishment worked. After a vomiting spell later that evening, Nancy emptied her plate at every meal, leaving no crumbs or bites behind. She did not openly rebel against her mother's rules, realizing her mother's power, which was a result of her father's frequent business travels. Nancy felt lonely; she would have wanted to bond with her father, but his absences kept him from being a regular family member. In addition, her younger sister, Susan, was their mother's favorite. The mother frequently cooked Susan's favorite dishes because they were also her favorite food items, and both made a big scene enjoying them. Nancy felt like an outsider. As she did not dare express her anger openly, she managed to get some secret satisfaction from silently criticizing her mother's plump figure. Inwardly, she judged her mother harshly for not being disciplined enough to keep a slim and trim figure.

Growing up emotionally detached from family members; while hiding her seething anger under a camouflage of obedience, Nancy's main source of reward was the unvoiced criticism of her mother. And the strong, silent criticism of overweight people remained with her for the rest of her life.

At Work

People with OCDP often do not attain the level of professional achievement that might be predicted on the basis of their talents and abilities, because their rigidity and stubbornness make them poor "team players" or supervisors.

OCPD usually interferes with interpersonal relationships, but it can make work functioning more efficient. It is not the job itself that is impacted by the disorder but rather the relationship with coworkers, or even employers, that might be strained.

The perfectionism and self-imposed high standards of performance that individuals with OCPD adopt for their lives can create stressful situations not only within their families but also in many work situations as their colleagues and supervisors become increasingly concerned about missed deadlines. They might be described as conscientious workers, but they often have difficulties finishing projects on time because they must follow their own step-by-step procedures or repeatedly revise what they are working on. And unless they can control the quality of what others do, they have problems delegating work to others.

People with OCPD are known for being very controlling and bossy toward other people, especially subordinates. Their insistence that there is only one way (their way) to perform a chore or do a job often leads to strained work situations and may result in an attitude of passive-aggressiveness in their coworkers and subordinates. They cannot allow anyone—including themselves—to bend any rules. Their attitudes toward their own superiors or supervisors, however, depend on whether they respect them as authorities. Individuals with OCPD are usually very courteous to those superiors they respect, but they can be quite resistant to or contemptuous of those they do not respect (Mind Disorders, 2018).

Work environments may reward OCPD individuals' conscientiousness and attention to detail, but they do not show much spontaneity or imagination. In fact, when immediate action is required, they may feel paralyzed and overwhelmed by trying to make decisions without concrete guidelines. As they expect their colleagues to stick to detailed rules, they often perform poorly in jobs that require flexibility and the ability to compromise. Even when individuals with OCPD are behind schedule, delegating work to others makes them feel uncomfortable because the others may not do the job "properly." Often, people with OCPD get so lost in the finer parts of a task that they can't see the bigger picture.

Up Close

Betty did not like surprises; she needed to know the plans for the day so she could perform her activities according to plan and as perfectly as possible. Directions had to be simple and clear so they could be followed to the letter. There was little or no room for change. Consistency was her security blanket, which she was not willing to surrender. Some of Betty's friends thought her career choice was a poor choice—whoever heard of an obsessive-compulsive beautician? Beauticians were thought to be style-changing free spirits. They had to keep up with the fashion trends of the day. Betty agreed; she knew she had to accommodate changing times and their expression in changing hairstyles, but within the changing expressions, certain rules still prevailed. For instance, each step in the process of haircutting, styling, and coloring needed to be performed with perfection, just as was the case with every step in other aspects of the beautifying process. And Betty had learned each step to perfection.

To cope with alterations required by the changing fashion trends, Betty surrounded her work station with photographs of models whose hairstyles reflected the current trends. Those of Betty's customers who did not have their own style ideas were asked to choose from among the photographs.

Over time, the customers of the beauty parlor were divided into three groups. One group insisted on being served by Betty with a hairstyle they had felt comfortable with for years. The second group also appreciated Betty's work, but they were willing to make their choice of hairstyle from the photographs. The customers in the third group refused to get close to Betty. They were the people who wanted to be creative and request changes while their heads were engaged in the beautifying process. Overall, it worked out well because there was enough work left for the other beauticians, and Betty's customers could rest assured they would leave the beauty parlor looking exactly the same as they had on previous visits.

In Relationships

Individuals with OCPD often experience a moderate level of professional success, but their relationships with friends, spouses, or children may be strained due to their combination of emotional detachment and controlling behaviors.

Interpersonally, the person with OCPD is capable of concern and mutuality in relationships but may encounter difficulty living with a new roommate or spouse. Family members of people with this disorder often feel criticized and controlled by individuals with OCPD. Expressions of tender feelings make people with OCPD feel uncomfortable, and they tend to avoid relatives and friends who are more emotionally expressive.

Their strict and ungenerous approach to life limits their ability to relax, and they find it difficult to release their need for control. Many

OCPD sufferers bring office work along on vacations without consideration for their spouses' disappointment. Not surprisingly, this combination of characteristics puts a strain on their interpersonal relationships and can lead to a lonely existence.

With OCPD patients, perception of their own and others' actions and beliefs tends to be polarized into "right" or "wrong," with little or no margin between the two. This could produce strain on interpersonal relationships with occasional frustration leading to disinhibition, which can turn into anger and even varying degrees of violence (Villemarette-Pittman, Stanford, Greve, Houston, & Mathias, 2004).

Up Close

Bruno had a difficult time getting used to living by himself again. A little more than two months ago, Cynthia had moved out of their house into a lovely condominium a couple of miles away. It was the second marriage for both of them. Bruno, at 39 years of age, experienced a mixture of emotions: sadness about Cynthia's move mixed in with anger and disappointment as he walked through the half-empty house, stopping at the twins' bedroom. The girls lived with their mother but spent some weekends and vacations with him and Cynthia. How would he explain this change of living separately but still being married to each other to his daughters?

Cynthia's reason for the move was—as she stated it—"Let's see if we can save this marriage."

"How can you think of saving a marriage by moving out?" Bruno asked in surprise.

"I feel like your rules—that everything needs to be done in a certain way, and every item needs to be put in its defined space—are strangling my love for you. Instead of looking forward to our being together after work and on weekends, I find myself worrying if everything is in its right place," Cynthia explained.

"I only want what's best and most efficient in our busy lives," Bruno defended himself, indicating that he knew what was best for both of them.

"Living in two different places would eliminate my worry and your concerns. We could just visit with each other and enjoy each other's company without any other responsibility about how the household is functioning," Cynthia explained again.

Even if Bruno accepted this physical separation, Cynthia knew that a lot still depended on Bruno's behavior. Would he be able to be in her condominium without changing some of the furniture or decorative items? Would he be able to relax in her place to the point that both of them could enjoy the other's company? She hoped so, and she was willing to give this new experiment plenty of time.

Theory and Research

A study, partly funded by the National Institutes of Health, investigated the biological basis for both compulsive and impulsive personality disorders (Stein et al., 1996). Along with other study participants, the study compared the lives of two men, who resembled one another in several significant ways; behavioral as well as biochemical parallels were identified. It was found that the participants had chemical differences in their neurotransmitters that distinguished them from the general population. The observed chemical differences correlated with the number of compulsive traits exhibited in their lives. Focusing on the neurotransmitter serotonin, the researchers noted an indication that the patients' destructive behavior patterns were connected with abnormalities in their serotonin levels. Whether such biological differences are present at birth or if people's experience also cause chemical changes in the brain is unknown.

A 2014 study about differences between OCPD and OCD found that samples afflicted with OCPD, regardless of the presence of comorbid OCD, are more rigid in behavior and have greater delayed gratification than either those suffering from OCD or healthy control samples (Pinto, 2014). Delayed gratification is a measure of self-control, expressing the person's capacity to suppress the impulse to pursue more immediate gratification in order to gain greater rewards in the future.

Recent studies using *DSM-IV* criteria persistently reported high rates of OCPD in persons with OCD, with an approximate range of 23 percent to 32 percent in individuals with OCD. Some data suggest a possible specificity in the link between OCD and OCPD. OCPD rates are consistently higher in individuals with OCD than in healthy population controls using *DSM-IV* criteria (Pinto, Eisen, Mancebo, & Rasmussen, 2008).

While individuals with OCD are able to realize that their unwanted thoughts and ideas are unreasonable, people with OCPD are convinced that their way is the right and best way. This is a reason people with OCPD don't believe they need treatment. They believe that if everyone else conformed to their strict rules, everything would be fine.

Significant similarities overlap between OCPD and Asperger's syndrome (Gillberg & Billstedt, 2000), including the list-making, inflexible adherence to rules, and obsessive aspects of Asperger's syndrome.

However, Asperger's syndrome can be distinguished from OCPD by affective behaviors, more impaired social skills, difficulties with theory of mind (a general capacity to consider others' beliefs), and intense intellectual interests—for instance, an ability to recall every aspect of a hobby (Fitzgerald & Corvin, 2001). A 2009 study involving adult autistic participants revealed that 40 percent of those diagnosed with Asperger's syndrome met the diagnostic requirements for a comorbid OCPD diagnosis (Hofvander et al., 2009).

A consistent linkage between OCPD and eating disorders, especially anorexia nervosa, has been observed. Various studies have reported different incidence rates of OCPD among eating disorders. This may in part reflect differences in the methodology used in different studies, as well as the difficulties of diagnosing personality disorders (Halmi, 2005a).

Regardless of the prevalence of OCPD among eating disordered samples, OCPD's presence and overcontrolled quality seem to be positively correlated with a range of complications in eating disorders, as opposed to impulsive features (those linked with histrionic personality disorder), which predict better outcomes from treatment (Lilenfeld, 2006). Predictions with comorbid OCPD include more severe anorexic symptoms, worse remission rates (Crane, 2007), and the presence of aggravating behaviors, such as compulsive exercising.

A spectrum of childhood traits, reflecting obsessive-compulsive personality in adult women with eating disorders, was examined retrospectively to assess the predictive value of the traits for developing eating disorders (Anderluh, Tchanturia, Rabe-Hesketh, & Treasure, 2003). The study included 44 women with anorexia nervosa, 28 women with bulimia nervosa, and 28 healthy female comparison subjects. All were assessed with an interview instrument asking them to recall whether they had experienced some types of childhood behavior indicative of traits associated with OCPD. In addition, the subjects completed a self-report inventory of OCD symptoms. Results showed that childhood OCPD traits had a high predictive value for the development of eating disorders. Those subjects with eating disorders who reported perfectionism and rigidity in childhood had significantly higher rates of OCPD and OCD comorbidity later in life, compared with eating disorder subjects who did not report those traits. It was concluded that traits reflecting OCPD evident in childhood appear to be significant risk factors for the development of eating disorders. They may represent markers of a broader phenotype for a specific subgroup of patients with anorexia nervosa.

Another important OCPD trait, perfectionism, has been linked with anorexia nervosa for decades. Anorexic women's incessant striving for thinness is a manifestation of this trait, which features an insistence upon meeting unattainably high standards of performance. In addition to perfectionism, other OCPD traits have been noted in the childhoods of individuals with eating disorders in significantly greater frequency than among control samples, including among their sisters who were not affected. Similar to individuals afflicted with OCPD, people with anorexia and bulimia also appear to have a greater need for order and symmetry in their activities and environments, something that is also observed in connection with OCD (Serpell, 2002). Individuals afflicted with eating disorders seem to be less likely to develop the multiobject obsessions and compulsions of those with classic OCD, who generally self-report symptoms related to a multitude of themes. In contrast, the symptoms of both, people with anorexia and bulimia, seem to be more restricted to symmetry and orderliness concerns, similar to what has been observed in samples afflicted with comorbid OCPD and OCD rather than just OCD (Lochner et al., 2011).

In a study involving two samples—one with both restrictive anorexia and OCD and another with OCD without an eating disorder—those with comorbid anorexia and OCD were more likely to be diagnosed with OCPD than those from the sample with OCD only (38.1% vs. 8.7%; Halmi, 2005b). Another sample including anorexic bingers and normal-weight bulimics showed that all three eating-disordered groups were more likely to develop symptoms surrounding order and symmetry than the OCD-only group.

Inflexibility and overattention to detail, additional OCPD traits, have also been found in cognitive testing of anorexics. Compared to healthy controls, this group will display average to above average performance in tests requiring accuracy (Southgate, 2008) but poorly on tests requiring mental flexibility and the ability to integrate details of information into a bigger narrative (Van Autreve, 2013).

Both non-eating-disordered OCPD and anorexic study samples also shared the trait of increased self-control, that is, an above-average ability to delay gratification in the interest of a greater good to be received in the future (Steinglass, 2012).

A similar experiment involved four non-eating-disordered samples—one with OCPD only, another with OCD only, a third afflicted with both OCPD and OCD, and a sample of healthy controls. Delayed gratification was pronounced in the OCPD group only and not in the other samples. In fact, delayed gratification was highly correlated with the severity of OCPD. In other words, the greater the capacity to delay gratification in individuals afflicted with OCPD, the more impairing the disorder. Many psychiatric disorders—like substance abuse, for example—may involve impulse deregulation; OCPD and anorexia nervosa are the only disorders shown to bring about the opposite quality: excessive self-control (Pinto, 2014).

A close genetic link between OCPD and anorexia has been found in some family studies comparing three sets of women for a variety of psychiatric diagnoses. One group was suffering from the restricting type of anorexia nervosa, another from bulimia nervosa, and a control group of women without an eating disorder plus their respective relatives unaffected by eating disorders. A much higher incidence of OCPD was found among anorexics and their relatives than in the control samples and their own relatives. In addition, the rates of OCPD among relatives of anorexics with that personality disorder and those without it were about the same. This indicates a shared familial transmission of anorexia and OCPD. Bulimics and their relatives did not show elevated rates of OCPD (Lilenfeld, 1998).

A similarly intended study also reported much higher incidence of OCPD among relatives of restrictive anorexics than among relatives of a normal control group. Along with diagnoses of OCD and generalized anxiety disorder, OCPD was the one that most clearly distinguished between the two groups (Strober, 2007).

Comparing the levels of psychosocial functioning in patients with schizotypal, borderline, avoidant, or obsessive-compulsive personality disorder and patients with major depressive disorder and no personality disorder, a study revealed that OCPD was associated with the least overall functional impairment among the personality disorders (Skodol et al., 2002).

Although a defining feature of personality disorder is an enduring pattern of inner experience and behavior that is stable over time, some studies have demonstrated considerable diagnostic instability of personality disorders, even over short intervals. In order to determine the stability of impairment in psychosocial functioning in patients with four different personality disorders in contrast to patients with major depressive disorder only (MDD and no PD) over a 2-year period, 600 treatment-seeking or treated patients were recruited and assigned to one of five diagnostic groups (schizotypal personality disorder, borderline personality disorder, avoidant personality disorder, obsessive-compulsive personality disorder, or major depressive disorder with no personality disorder), based on the results of semistructured interview assessments and self-report measures. Results obtained at baseline and at three follow-up assessments showed significant improvement in psychosocial functioning in only three of seven domains of functioning, and this was largely the result of improvements in the MDD-no-PD group. Patients with OCPD or BPD showed no improvement in functioning overall. Impairment in social relationships seemed stable in patients with personality disorders (Skodol et al., 2005).

Comparing the two Skodol et al. studies, it is interesting to note that in the earlier (2002) study, individuals with OCPD showed the least overall functional impairment among the personality disorders, whereas in the later (2005) study, OCPD (and most personality disorders) showed no improvement in functioning; the main source in improvement was within the MDD patients. Thus, both studies seem to attest to the stability of functional impairment within OCPD.

Using attachment theory as a framework to elucidate the interpersonal dysfunction characteristic of OCPD, a study assessed attachment security and personality disorders in adult inpatients with severe mental illness. It was found that the group of individuals with OCPD (n = 61) showed greater attachment avoidance than the control group (n = 61). The avoidance was predominantly apparent with fearful attachment, the most insecure attachment style. The findings confirmed the severity of impairment in interpersonal functioning and attachment avoidance, which is characteristic of people with OCPD. The results suggest that interpersonal functioning constitutes a viable treatment target, along with more classical features of OCPD such as perfectionism and obsessiveness in task performance (Wiltgen et al., 2015).

Another study with OCPD inpatients compared rates of clinically significant and reliable change in psychopathology and global functioning, prevalence of clinical deterioration, and rates of symptom remission among adult patients with OCPD (n = 52) and well-matched inpatients with other personality disorders (n = 56) and patients with no personality disorder (n = 53). The results revealed that the OCPD patients were admitted to treatment with higher rates of depression, anxiety, difficulty with emotion regulation, and nonacceptance of emotional experience than the inpatient control groups. While OCPD patients responded to treatment at a similar rate as did the inpatient controls, they experienced lower rates of anxiety remission upon discharge. Post hoc analyses indicate that individuals meeting OCPD stubbornness and rigidity criteria were nine times more likely to report moderate to severe anxiety at discharge. In conclusion, the study showed that overall, OCPD inpatients benefit from intensive multimodal psychiatric treatment, but upon discharge, they experience more anxiety than patients without personality disorders (Smith, Shepard, Wiltgen, Rufino, & Fowler, 2017).

Treatment

Learning to find satisfaction in life through close relationships with others and recreational outlets, instead of only through work-related activities, can significantly enrich the OCPD patient's life. Specific training in relaxation techniques may help OCPD patients who have the so-called "Type A" characteristics of competitiveness, time urgency, and preoccupation with work. However, the development of a therapeutic alliance with an OCPD patient may be difficult because the patient enters therapy with a powerful need to control the situation (and the therapist), a reluctance to trust others, and a tendency to doubt just about everything connected with the therapy situation. The therapist needs to be alert to the patient's defenses against genuine change. Gaining a level of commitment to the therapeutic process from the patient is a difficult task for any therapist.

Treatment for OCPD includes psychotherapy, cognitive behavioral therapy, behavior therapy, or self-help. Cognitive analytic therapy is an effective form of behavior therapy. But treatment can be complicated if individuals don't accept that they have OCPD, or if they believe that their thoughts or behaviors are correct and therefore should not be changed.

For many years, medications for OCPD and other personality disorders were considered to be ineffective because they do not directly affect the underlying causes of the disorder. But more recent studies indicate that treatment with specific drugs may be a useful adjunct to psychotherapy. While medication alone is generally not indicated for this disorder, selective serotonin reuptake inhibitors (SSRIs) may be useful in addition to psychotherapy by helping individuals to be less bogged down with minor details, and it may also lessen their rigidity and compulsiveness. Although this method of symptom control may not "cure" the underlying personality disorder, medication does enable some OCPD patients to function with less distress.

Long-term psychotherapy focusing directly on the patient's rigid beliefs and inflexible behavior has been observed to be helpful in treating obsessive-compulsive patients. Although antianxiety drugs have been used with OCPD, caution is advised because of the chronicity of the disorder, which may lead to medication dependency.

Individuals with OCPD are three times more likely to receive individual psychotherapy than people with major depressive disorder (Bender et al., 2006). There are few large-scale studies involving people afflicted with OCPD, but reports suggest that treatment can help, leading to greater insight into how someone's OCPD symptoms affect others. Often it takes the threat of the loss of a relationship or job to motivate people with OCPD to seek treatment. If motivated to change, psychotherapy holds much promise (Van Noppen, 2010).

Because OCPD sufferers, unlike people with OCD, tend to view their compulsive behaviors as voluntary, they are in a better condition to consider change, especially as they come to fully recognize the personal and interpersonal costs of their disorder (Mind Disorders, 2018).

References

Anderluh, M. B., Tchanturia, K., Rabe-Hesketh, S., & Treasure, J. (2003). Childhood obsessive-compulsive personality traits in adult women with eating disorders: Defining a broader eating disorder phenotype. *Psychiatry Online*. doi:10.1176/appi.160.2.242

Bayer, L. (2000). *Personality disorders*. Philadelphia, PA: Chelsea House Publishers.

Bender, D., Skodol, A. E., Pagano, M. E., Dyck, I. R., Grilo, C. M., Shea, M. T., . . . Gunderson, J. G. (2006). Prospective assessment of treatment use by patients with personality disorders. *Psychiatric Service, 57*(2), 254–257.

Bressert, S. (2017). Obsessive-compulsive personality disorder. *Psych Central*. Retrieved February 21, 2018, from https://psychcentral.com/disorder/obsessive-compulsive personality disorder/

Crane, A. (2007). Are obsessive-compulsive personality traits associated with a poor outcome in anorexia nervosa? A systematic review of randomized controlled trials and naturalistic outcome studies. *International Journal of Eating Disorders, 40*(7), 581–588.

Fineberg, N. A., Sharma, P., Sivakumaran, T., Sahakian, B., & Chamberlain, S. (2007). Does obsessive-compulsive personality disorder belong within the obsessive-compulsive spectrum? *CNS Spectrum, 12*(6), 467–474, 477–482.

Fitzgerald, M., & Corvin, A. (2001). Diagnosis and differential diagnosis of Asperger syndrome. *Advances in Psychiatric Treatment, 7*(4), 310–318.

Foa, E. B., Kozak, M. J., Goodman, W. K., Hollander, E., Jenike, M. A., & Rasmussen, S. A. (1995). Obsessive compulsive disorder. *DSM-IV* field trial, *American Journal of Psychiatry, 152*, 90–96.

Gillberg, C., & Billstedt, E. (2000). Autism and Asperger syndrome: Coexistence with other clinical disorders. *Acta Psychiatrica Scandinavica, 102*(5), 321–330.

Grant, B. F., Hasin, D. S., Stinson, F. S., Dawson, D. A., Chou, S. P., Ruan, W. J., & Pickering, R. P. (2004). Prevalence, correlates, and disability of personality disorders in the United States: Results from the National Epidemiologic Survey on Alcohol and Related Conditions. *The Journal of Clinical Psychiatry, 65*(7), 948–958.

Halmi, K. A. (2005a). Obsessive-compulsive personality disorder and eating disorders. *Eating Disorders, 13*(1), 85–92.

Halmi, K. A. (2005b). The relation among perfectionism, obsessive-compulsive personality disorder and obsessive-compulsive disorder in individuals with eating disorders. *International Journal of Eating Disorders, 38*(4), 371–374.

Hofvander, B., Delorme, R., Chaste, P., Nyden, A., Wentz, E., Stahlberg, . . . Leboyer, M. (2009). Psychiatric and psychosocial problems in adults with normal-intelligence autism spectrum disorders. *BMC Psychiatry, 9*(1), 35.

Jefferys, D., & Moore, K. A. (2008). Pathological hoarding. *Australian Family Physician, 37*(4), 237–241.

Lilenfeld, L. (1998). A controlled family study of anorexia nervosa and bulimia nervosa: Psychiatric disorders in first-degree relatives and effects of proband comorbidity. *Archives of General Psychiatry, 55*(7), 603–610.

Lilenfeld, L. R. (2006). Eating disorders and personality: A methodological and empirical review. *Clinical Psychological Review, 26*, 299–320.

Lochner, C., Serebro, P., van der Merwe, L., Hemmings, S., Kinnear, C., Seedat, S., & Stein, D. J. (2011). Comorbid obsessive-compulsive personality disorder in obsessive-compulsive disorder (OCD): A marker of severity. *Progress in Neuro-Psychopharmacology & Biological Psychiatry, 35*(4), 1087–1092.

Millon, T. (2004). *Personality disorders in modern life*. Hoboken, NJ: John Wiley & Sons.

Mind Disorders. (2018). Obsessive-compulsive personality disorder. Retrieved February 26, 2018, from http://www.minddisorders.com /Ob-Ps/Obsessive-compulsive-personality-disorder.html

Pinto, A. (2014). Capacity to delay reward differentiates obsessive-compulsive disorder and obsessive-compulsive personality disorder. *Biological Psychiatry, 75*(8), 63–69.

Pinto, A., Eisen, J. L., Mancebo, M. C., & Rasmussen, S. A. (2008). Obsessive-compulsive personality disorder. In J. S. Abramowitz, D. McKay, & S. Taylor (Eds.), *Obsessive-compulsive disorder: Subtypes and spectrum conditions* (pp. 246–263). Cambridge, MA: Elsevier.

Reichborn-Kjennerud, T., Neale, M. C., Orstavik, R. C., Torgersen, S., Tambs, K., Roysamb, E., . . . Kendler, K. S. (2007). Genetic and environmental influences on dimensional representations of DSM-IV cluster C personality disorders: A population-based multivariate twin study. *Psychological Medicine, 37*(5), 645–653.

Salzman, L. (1968). *The obsessive personality: Origins, dynamics, and therapy*. New York, NY: Science House.

Samuel, D. B., & Griffin, S. A. (2015). Obsessive-compulsive personality disorder. *Wiley Online Library*. First published January 23, 2015. doi:10.1002/9781118625392.wbecp210

Serpell, L. (2002). Anorexia nervosa: Obsessive-compulsive disorder, obsessive-compulsive personality disorder, or neither? *Clinical Psychology Review, 22*(5), 647–669.

Skodol, A. E., Gunderson, J. G., McGlashan, T. H., Dyck, I. R., Stout, R. L., Bender, D. S., . . . Oldham, J. M. (2002). Functional impairment in patients with schizotypal, borderline, avoidant, or obsessive-compulsive personality disorder. *American Journal of Psychiatry, 159*(2), 276–283.

Skodol, A. E., Pagano, M. E., Bender, D. S., & Shea, M. T. (2005). Stability of functional impairment in patients with schizotypal, borderline, avoidant, or obsessive-compulsive personality disorder over two years. *Psychological Medicine, 35*(3), 443–451.

Smith, R., Shepard, C., Wiltgen, A., Rufino, K., & Fowler, J. C. (2017). Treatment outcomes for inpatients with obsessive-compulsive personality disorder: An open comparison trial. *Journal of Affective Disorders, 209*(February), 273–278.

Southgate, L. (2008). Information processing bias in anorexia nervosa. *Psychiatry Research, 160*(2), 221–227.

Stein, D., J., Trestman, R. L., Mitropoulou, V., Coccaro, E. F., Hollander, E., & Siever, L. J. (1996). Impulsivity and serotonergic function in compulsive personality disorder. *Journal of Neuropsychiatry and Clinical Neurosciences, 8*(4), 393–398.

Steinglass, J. (2012). Increased capacity to delay reward in anorexia nervosa. *Journal of the International Neuropsychological Society, 18*, 1–8.

Strober, M. (2007). The association of anxiety disorders and obsessive-compulsive personality disorder with anorexia nervosa: Evidence from a family study with discussion of nosological and neurodevelopmental implications. *International Journal of Eating Disorders, 40*, S46–S51.

Van Autreve, S. (2013). Do restrictive and bingeing/purging subtypes of anorexia nervosa differ on central coherence and set shifting? *European Eating Disorders Review, 21*(4), 308–314.

Van Noppen, B. (2010). *Obsessive-compulsive personality disorder (OCPD).* Boston, MA: International OCD Foundation (IOCDF).

Villemarette-Pittman, N. R., Stanford, M., Greve, K., Houston, R., & Mathias, C. (2004). Obsessive-compulsive personality disorder and behavioral disinhibition. *The Journal of Psychology, 138*(1), 5–22.

Wiltgen, A., Adler, H., Smith, R., Rufino, K., Frazier, C., Shepard, C., . . . Fowler, J. C. (2015). Attachment insecurity and obsessive-compulsive personality disorder among inpatients with serious mental illness. *Journal of Affective Disorders, 174,* 411–415.

CHAPTER 8

Paranoid Personality Disorder

Symptoms, Diagnosis, and Incidence

A pattern of pervasive distrust and suspiciousness of others constitutes the essential feature of paranoid personality disorder (PPD), according to *DSM-5*. The motives of others are generally interpreted by people with PPD to be malevolent. Beginning in early adulthood, this pattern is present in a variety of contexts.

Even in the absence of evidence to support their negative expectations, there is always the assumption that people will exploit them, harm them, or deceive them. People with PPD do not need evidence to firmly believe that others are plotting against them and will attack them suddenly without reason. Unjustified doubts about the loyalty or trustworthiness of their friends and acquaintances preoccupy the minds of individuals with this disorder. But this is not a psychotic disorder.

Their overriding pervasive suspiciousness does not allow individuals with PPD to confide in or become close to others because they are afraid that whatever information they share with others will be used against them. Even offers of help from others may be viewed by the individual with PPD as an act of criticism, indicating that the individual is not competent to take care of him- or herself.

With all the distrust and negative interpretations of others' behavior and intentions, it is not surprising that people afflicted with PPD are unwilling to forgive others their perceived insults and bear grudges for long periods of time. Anger and jealousy are common reactions to their expected and/or misinterpreted evaluation of those around them.

Individuals with PDP are suspicious of people in virtually all situations in their personal and professional lives.

Because of their lack of trust in others, individuals with PPD have an excessive need for self-sufficiency and autonomy. They want to be in control not only over their own destinies but also over those around them. This excessive need for control leads to stressful situations in their personal lives and especially in work situations. In addition, thinly hidden, unrealistic grandiose fantasies related to issues of power and rank often lead to the development of negative stereotypes of others, particularly those from groups different from their own.

In response to stress, individuals with this disorder may experience very brief psychotic episodes, and in some instances, PPD may develop into delusional disorder or become a precursor to the paranoid type of schizophrenia.

Data from the National Epidemiologic Survey on Alcohol and Related Conditions suggest a prevalence of PPD of 4.4 percent, while an estimate based on a probability subsample from Part II of the National Comorbidity Survey Replication points to a prevalence of 2.3 percent. In clinical samples, PPD appears to be more commonly diagnosed in males than in females. The estimate of people afflicted with this disorder within the general population ranges from 0.5 to 2.5 percent, again, with males more commonly afflicted than females (Internet Mental Health, 2018). Interestingly, another estimate suggested that nearly 4 percent of the general population seems to struggle with the disorder, but with women reporting the problem more frequently than men (Grant et al., 2004). It is not known whether the changes are due to elapsed time or whether there are other reasons for the discrepancy.

PPD often first appears in childhood or adolescence. It may manifest itself as solitary behavior, poor relations with peers, social anxiety, and hypersensitivity as well as underachievement in school, idiosyncratic fantasies, or peculiar thoughts and language. But it is not commonly diagnosed in childhood or adolescence, because in the developing individual, personality traits change with maturation. Generally, this disorder is not diagnosed when another psychotic disorder, such as schizophrenia or a bipolar or depressive disorder with psychotic features, has already been diagnosed in a person (Bressert, 2017).

The World Health Organization's *ICD-10* PPD classification includes expansive paranoid, fanatic, querulant, and sensitive PPD types but excludes delusional disorder and schizophrenia.

Timeline

1893   French psychiatrist V. Magnan distinguished between two categories of paranoid psychosis.

1905   Emil Kraepelin described a pseudo-querulous personality type, who is always ready to find a grievance.

1908   Eugen Bleuler described "contentious psychopathy."

1911   Freud related paranoid tendencies to the repudiation of latent homosexuality through projection.

1921   Kraepelin expanded his earlier description of a "fragile personality" and renamed it paranoid personality.

1924   Bleuler described the conditions "contentious psychopath" or "paranoid constitution" and emphasized the characteristic triad of suspiciousness, grandiosity, and feelings of persecution.

1927   Kretschmer emphasized the sensitive inner core of the paranoid-prone personality.

1940s Jaspers described "self-insecure personalities" bearing a close resemblance to paranoid personality disorder.

1950   Kurt Schneider described a condition of "fanatic psychopaths."

1961   Shepherd provided a thorough profile of paranoid personality disorder.

1965   Shapiro identified two types of paranoid personality: "furtive, constricted, apprehensively suspicious individuals and rigidly arrogant, more aggressively suspicious, megalomanic ones" (p. 54).

1981   Millon divided the features of paranoid personality into four categories (obdurate, fanatic, querulous, insular, and malignant paranoid subtypes).

History

Perhaps one of the earliest portrayals of PPD in the psychiatric literature was provided by the French psychiatrist V. Magnan in 1893 when he differentiated paranoid psychoses into two categories, "chronic delusional state of systematic evolution" and the "delusional states of the degenerates." He further divided the second category into three subtypes: paranoia associated with mental defect, chronic delusional states with a good long-term prognosis, and the delusional states of degeneracy. The third condition was characterized by sudden onset, clouded sensorium, affective coloring, and rapid remission. In Magnan's opinion, such short-lasting paranoid development had its foundation in a constitutional degeneracy or a "fragile personality" that exhibited idiosyncratic thinking, hypochondria, undue sensitivity, suspiciousness, and referential thinking (Akhtar, 1990).

Another description of a pseudo-querulous, self-absorbed, sensitive, irritable, obstinate, and litigious personality type was offered by Kraepelin in 1905, which he renamed paranoid personality in 1921. In his more detailed description, Kraepelin characterized such individuals as feeling unjustly treated by everyone and seeing themselves as the objects of hostility, interference, and oppression. Persons with paranoid personality were observed to be chronically irritable and behaving in a boastful, impatient, and obstinate manner. Kraepelin noted another contradiction in paranoid personalities: as they stubbornly hold on to their unusual beliefs and ideas, they frequently accept every piece of gossip as the truth. He further observed that paranoid personalities were often encountered in individuals who later developed paranoid psychosis. Certain traits, like suspiciousness and hostility, were considered by other writers to predispose people to developing delusional illnesses, such as "late paraphrenias" of old age (Bernstein, Useda, & Siever, 1995).

In describing conditions he called "contentious psychopathy" or "paranoid constitution," Bleuler (1908) emphasized the characteristic triad of suspiciousness, grandiosity, and feelings of persecution and the absence of real delusions in individuals afflicted with this condition. The sensitive inner core of the paranoid-prone personality was emphasized by Kretschmer (1927), explaining that these individuals feel shy and inadequate, but at the same time, they hold an attitude of entitlement. Their failures are attributed to the intrigues of others, but secretly, they blame their own inadequacy. There is a constant internal tension between feelings of self-importance and experiencing the world around them as unappreciative and humiliating (Akhtar, 1990).

During the 1940s the German phenomenologist Jaspers gave a description of "self-insecure personalities" that bears a close resemblance to PPD. Jaspers's (1949) explanation was that these individuals lead a life of inner humiliation resulting from outside experiences and their interpretation of them.

Using the term "psychopath" as the equivalent of the current term "personality disorder," Kurt Schneider in 1950 described a group of individuals under the designation "fanatic psychopaths." The fanatic psychopaths consisted of two types, one being combative and the other eccentric. Individuals of the combative type exhibited quarrelsome and litigious behavior, complaining bitterly, and seeking justice. Eccentric-type psychopaths were passive and secretive but harbored suspicious and false assumptions about others. Similarly, Leonhard in 1959 emphasized that paranoid individuals attribute any of their failures to the ill will of others, while at the same time overvaluing their own abilities and competencies.

In addition to Shepherd's (1961) provision of a thorough profile of PPD, Polatin in 1975 suggested a description of individuals with paranoid personality disorder as rigid, suspicious, watchful, self-centered and selfish and added that these individuals also tend to be arrogant, secretive, critical, humorless, and inconsiderate. These characteristics are often covered by a facade of affability, which may shatter easily when there is a difference of opinion to disclose the underlying mistrust, authoritarianism, and hate.

Textbook descriptions of paranoid personality during the 1970s appeared to be relatively uniform, but some provided greater clarity than others. Two types of paranoid personality were distinguished by others: the sensitive type, which was considered to be characterized by subdued resentment and cynicism, and the querulant paranoid type, which was expressed in open defiance and litigiousness (Hamilton, 1974). Another frequently noted aspect was what seemed to be contradictions in the paranoid makeup, such as the paranoid individual's "contradictory pride and lack of self-confidence" (Slater & Roth, 1977, p. 149). Similarly, the coexistence of feelings of superiority and inferiority were noted (Salzman, 1974) as well as the paranoid individual's overt stubbornness and hidden self-doubt (Stanton, 1978).

PPD did not receive much attention during the 1980s. Theodore Millon was probably the most significant contributor of this decade. In 1981 he divided the features of PPD into four categories: (1) behavioral characteristics of vigilance, abrasive irritability, and counterattack; (2) complaints indicating oversensitivity, social isolation, and mistrust; (3) the dynamics of denying personal insecurities, attributing them to others and self-inflation through grandiose fantasies; and (4) coping style of detesting dependence and hostile distancing of oneself from others (Akhtar, 1990).

Like other investigators, Millon noted that "the confidence and pride of paranoids cloak but a hollow shell . . . [and their] . . . arrogant pose of autonomy rests on insecure footings" (1981, p. 383).

Paranoid personality disorder had been included in all previous versions of the *DSM* and is currently listed in the *DSM-5*.

Development and Causes

Paranoid personality disorder may be observable as early as in childhood or adolescence with poor peer relationships, social anxiety, hypersensitivity, idiosyncratic fantasies, and peculiar thoughts and language on the part of the sufferer. Even as children, they may appear to be "odd" or eccentric and may attract teasing.

A strong connection between sadomasochism and paranoid psychopathology was noted by Freud, pointing out that individuals who harbor unconscious beating fantasies often develop sensitivity and irritability toward persons whom they can include in the class of fathers. In his later writings, Freud (1922) mentioned three factors that were important in the genesis of paranoid pathology: an initial aggressive disposition, early experiences of threat to survival, and an aggression toward the mother during the preoedipal phase of development.

In Kleinian thinking, the paranoid-schizoid position is considered to be the developmental basis for all severe character pathology; it is the earliest constellation of infantile object relations. Characteristic of the first six months of life, this position is capable of later activation and may become a habitual personality style. Threatened from within by inborn aggression, the infantile ego resorts to projection that, in turn, creates persecutory anxiety, which is defended against by splitting, denial, and primitive idealization (Klein, 1932). Through splitting, the "good" and "bad" objects are kept apart; the good objects will be introjected and identified with by the individual, whereas the bad objects are projected onto others.

The role of the external environment in the development of paranoid traits was emphasized by Winnicott (1953), who suggested that the infant experiences any interference with his being as a nuisance. Birth itself is a template for disturbance. Unless the mother—in addition to satisfying the infant's basic needs—provides an unobtrusive presence in the background where the infant can somehow process the various experiences, anxiety, inner withdrawal, and diminution of psychic freedom will follow. Later on such a child will display suspiciousness, lack of playfulness, and preoccupation with fantasies of cruelty. Social isolation, persecutory dreams, overtly paranoid fantasies, and sadomasochistic sexual concerns will be added to the clinical picture with the onset of adolescence.

Erikson (1950) also thought that paranoid trends had their genesis in overwhelming frustration during infancy, which would impede the development of basic trust. The lack of confidence that develops is followed by increasing helplessness, pessimism, and feelings of shame and doubt.

Other authors (e.g., Cameron, 1963) explain that many individuals with PPD had actually been treated cruelly during early childhood and, as a result, internalized sadistic attitudes toward themselves and others. Similarly, it was observed that paranoid individuals often had grown up in families with overt cruelty and bickering between parents. Thus, a markedly sadomasochistic family atmosphere, often focusing on parents' marital infidelity, can be expected to set the stage for the development of the child's own sadism. Similarly, Jacobson (1971) observed that paranoid individuals had grown up in families that expressed cruel and arguing behaviors, as mentioned by Cameron and others.

Another opinion was expressed in the suggestion that paranoid personality was actually a subtype of narcissistic personality. The fundamental dynamic issue in paranoid personalities was thought to be their powerful unconscious longing for a reunion with the infantile parental objects (Bursten, 1973). Such longing was thought to stir up homosexual and incestuous fears as well as a dread of the dissolution of the self.

An association of paranoid personality with borderline personality organization or a "lower-level" character pathology was suggested by Kernberg (1975). Superego integration seems to be minimal at this point in the character organization, and the function of the ego is impaired. Kernberg also pointed out that narcissistic and PPD features may coexist. When that is the case, the decision regarding the dominant character constellation depends on the quality of prevalent object relations. While the paranoid individual's characteristics include being aloof, cold, and suspicious, they do not include the envy and exploitation demonstrated by narcissistic individuals.

Psychoanalytic views include Freud's attention to—among others—three important factors in the genesis of paranoid pathology, such as an initial aggressive disposition, actual early experiences of threat to survival, and aggression toward the mother during the preoedipal phase of development, while Melanie Klein (1932) regarded the "paranoid-schizoid position" as the earliest developmental constellation of infantile object relations. Psychosocial theories point to parental modeling and implicate projection of negative internal feelings, whereas cognitive theorists believe that the disorder is a result of an underlying belief that other people are unfriendly in combination with a lack of self-awareness (Beck & Freeman, 1990).

PPD is found more frequently among families in which close relatives have chronic schizophrenia than in the general population, suggesting the importance of heredity. The National Institute of Mental Health reports that PPD is found more often in families with a history of psychotic disorder like schizophrenia, indicating genetic factors; however, the individual's upbringing and experience are significant factors in determining the onset of the illness, according to most psychologists (Bayer, 2000).

The ultimate paranoid picture in adulthood is considered to be the result of a complex interplay of innate disposition, actual threats to survival during childhood, impaired object relations, and subsequent structural defects and defensive elaborations (Blum, 1981).

Effects and Costs

Although people with PPD are usually unable to acknowledge their own negative feelings toward others, they do not generally lose touch with reality.

Considering the fact that the main characteristic of paranoid personality disorder is a pattern of pervasive distrust and suspiciousness of others, combined with self-centered, critical, and arrogant behaviors, it is not difficult to understand that the greatest impact of the disorder will be in the afflicted individuals' interactions with others. As paranoid individuals remain distant in social interactions because of their distrust of others' motivations, those others involved in the situation may feel uncomfortable or offended by the aloof, critical, and often self-aggrandizing attitudes of those diagnosed with PPD.

In addition, the observed discrepancies between the inner world of people with PPD and their outer persona may be confusing to others around them. The condition seems to be characterized by several aspects, such as a profound mistrust with naive gullibility, hidden inferiority with arrogant demandingness, internal sensitivity with apparent emotional coldness, and hypervigilant attention with failure to comprehend the whole picture. Unable to understand these contradictions, others around them may refrain from getting to know the paranoid individual.

Therefore, the characteristics associated with PPD may produce a life with varying degrees of social isolation for those afflicted with the disorder. Even within romantic relationships, as well as within the circle of family life, intimacy and emotional closeness are usually lacking as paranoid individuals are reluctant to confide in others. Furthermore, their exaggerated need for self-sufficiency (brought on by their general distrust of others) will prevent paranoid individuals from seeking or requesting help—even if they desperately need the help. They distance themselves even from those who are truly concerned and interested in helping.

In response to stress, individuals with PPD can experience very brief psychotic episodes, lasting minutes to hours. If long-lasting, the disorder may develop into delusional disorder or schizophrenia. There is also a greater-than-average risk of experiencing major depressive disorder, agoraphobia, social anxiety disorder, obsessive-compulsive disorder, or alcohol and substance-related disorders for people with PPD.

Individuals with PPD may have other conditions that can feed into their PPD. Depression and anxiety, for instance, can affect a person's mood. Mood changes then can make PPD sufferers more likely to feel paranoid and isolated (Martel, 2017).

Eventually, PPD leads to considerable distress as it impairs the sufferer's function and success in social and professional settings; however, this may not happen until the person reaches his or her 40s or later (Healthy Place, 2016).

In Society

When considering the symptoms characteristic of PPD, it is not difficult to understand that persons afflicted with this disorder have difficulties getting along with others. Their suspiciousness, hypervigilance, sarcasm, self-centeredness, and inability to accept criticism or others' opinions give rise to stressful situations within families and among friends, neighbors, and coworkers. Their distrust of others often induces them to seek control over others. In spite of often being very critical of others, they do not accept criticism of themselves, and they do not tolerate ambiguities. The suspiciousness they experience most of the time may lead individuals suffering from PPD to develop negative stereotypes about others, which can express itself in racial, ethnic, or religious prejudice.

Their combative and suspicious nature may elicit a hostile response in other people, which the paranoid individuals then use to confirm their original negative expectations. They will not confide in people—even if they prove to be trustworthy—for fear of being exploited or betrayed. Their frequent misinterpretations of others' harmless comments and behaviors will build up and lead them to harbor unfounded resentment for an unreasonable length of time (Psychology Today, 2018).

People with PPD may behave in hostile or stubborn ways and may use sarcasm, which often elicits a hostile response from others—which, in turn, may seem to confirm their original suspiciousness (Martel, 2017).

At times a facade of affability may hide the rigid, critical, arrogant, and humorless attitudes of those suffering from PPD, but when there is a difference of opinion, the facade shatters, exposing the underlying mistrust and authoritarianism and allowing rage to reign.

These individuals' reduced capacity for meaningful emotional involvement and the pattern of their isolated withdrawals may lend a quality of schizoid isolation to their lives.

Up Close

Life with Tom was not easy; Harriet had learned over the years that Tom's suspiciousness knew no end. He always explained his unrelenting hypervigilance with the lessons he had learned in his professional life as an insurance adjuster. In his experience, everybody exaggerated any damage done to them, at other times accusing others of causing an accident or dangerous situation that had actually been their fault. Harriet was sad that they had no friends in the neighborhood. Although she was a friendly person, no neighbor woman invited Harriet for coffee or any kind of neighborhood meeting.

Tom's outward expressions of distrust, the high fence around his property with the big gate and "no trespassing" signs, the always tightly closed garage door, and the bright lights at night kept most people away. In fact, when walking along the neighborhood streets, people would cross over to the other side before coming to Tom's property. There was a constant battle with the company that had the contract for the neighborhood's garbage collection. A thrown or dented garbage can inspired a written complaint to the company, with a copy sent to the mayor's office.

On Halloween evening, Tom would sometimes wash his car in the driveway, discouraging any children from coming up and asking for treats because they knew they might well be hit by a stream of cold water. When the car did not need washing, Tom sat on the front porch with a rifle in his lap. He said it was not loaded, but nobody tried to take his word for it. However, on some Halloween nights, Tom paid a price for his hostility when a few of the older children, armed with raw eggs and ripe tomatoes, attacked his house late at night. They were never caught, and it did not happen every year, but it was enough to keep Tom's suspicion and hostile behavior going.

Over the years, Harriet had learned to deal with Tom's lack of trust in her own way. As she did not hold a job—Tom disapproved of women working in close proximity to men—she liked to go shopping when her children were in high school. But Tom did not approve of shopping beyond the food shopping for the family's meals, either. To avoid

arguments, Harriet devised her own little schemes. One of her maneu-
vers was to chop up onions and bacon in a frying pan before leaving on
her shopping trip. Shortly before Tom's return from work, Harriet raced
home, exchanged her coat for a pretty apron, and turned the stove on
full blast to fill the house with the smell of bacon and onions, as if she
had been sweating all day over the stove. When Tom opened the door,
Harriet greeted him, inviting him to sit down and relax with a cup of
coffee (previously prepared) and tell her about his day while she put
the "finishing touches" on their dinner. It worked for many decades
until Tom retired from his job. He never found out why he drank cof-
fee before dinner, although his daughter Jennifer knew; her mother had
told her.

At Work

In many life settings, but especially in competitive work settings, people with PPD are preoccupied with trustworthiness, which they usually
find lacking in their colleagues, subordinates, and bosses. In addition,
their hypervigilance in scrutinizing the actions of others, combined with
their hostile, aloof, and secretive behaviors, gives rise to an unfriendly,
stressful, and mutually suspicious work atmosphere. Their lack of trust
in others leads to an excessive need to be self-sufficient and the strong
desire to have control over those around them (Bressert, 2017). Combined with their inability to accept criticism, these characteristics will
not work well with members of work teams. As they overvalue their
own abilities, paranoid individuals are ambitious, driven, and extremely
sensitive to criticism. Their fears of betrayal are often counterbalanced
by grandiose fantasies and obsessions with power and rank, which may
lead them to expect special privileges. When those expectations remain
unfulfilled, colleagues are blamed for unfair competition, and supervisors may be suspected of acting with malevolent intentions toward the
paranoid personality.

Despite the chronic anxiety many paranoid individuals experience,
they retain a sufficient amount of unimpaired ego functions, such as
sharpness of observation, a tendency toward hair-splitting, and a rich
vocabulary. Many are eloquent speakers, but their primitive defense
operations center around splitting, denial, and projective identifica-
tion. Their defenses remain infiltrated with disavowed drive deriva-
tives, and paranoid individuals unconsciously gain some sadistic
pleasure in situations that they consciously register as only persecutory (Heimann, 1952).

Up Close

At 6:00 p.m., Bruce decided that he would have just enough time to go through his coworker's desk to check on the secret work papers Paul had taken from him and copied before placing them back in the left bottom drawer of Bruce's desk. Bruce could tell that the papers had been moved and arranged differently from the way he kept them. The cleaning crew would arrive around 7:30 p.m. All the employees on this floor seemed to have left for the day. Bruce was determined to not only retrieve the copies Paul had made but also to leave a small mousetrap under some sheets of paper in Paul's drawer. With any luck, Paul might get his finger snapped in the trap. If that did not happen, the presence of the trap would tell Paul that his crime had been detected. Bruce hoped that this would happen during working hours when Bruce and some of their coworkers could witness the scene.

Bruce was proud of the level of his intellectual abilities, and he was convinced that his colleagues envied him and wanted him to fail in the special project that had been assigned to him. This was his chance to confront everyone with his intelligence and capability. He was about to design and work out a sophisticated solution to the new project. Everybody would take notice of him. But it was not easy to protect his brainchild from the curiosity and envy of his colleagues. They talked about him behind his back and made fun of him because he had not achieved the doctoral degree that most of them claimed to hold. This was a sore subject for Bruce. After a very promising start in graduate school, he was dismissed from the university before he could earn a Ph.D. degree in electronic engineering. The reason for the dismissal was that Bruce had accused some of his classmates of stealing his ideas and using some of them in their own papers. Unfortunately, already distrustful of most people, Bruce was easy to anger, and he expressed his negative feelings in a somewhat explosive manner. According to Bruce, the two accused students had been able to hear when Bruce told his only remaining friend and classmate about his ideas and discoveries.

The results of the investigation did not reveal any evidence supporting Bruce's suspicions, and, in turn, the two accused graduate students complained to the president of the university. The result was Bruce's immediate dismissal with the warning that if he attempted to enter another university, the reason for his dismissal would be communicated to that university.

His future was ruined, and, not surprisingly, his suspicions and hostile vigilance grew in frequency and strength. Unfortunately, at the same time, he craved acknowledgment and praise for his intellectual abilities, and from time to time, he disclosed some of his ideas to those around him. However, with or without praise from those who heard about his greatness, it also reinforced his suspiciousness and feelings of persecution, because now that people knew about his specialness, they would soon dislike and punish him for it.

In Relationships

In a study of morbid jealousy, a detailed profile of PPD was provided by Shepherd in 1961. These individuals constantly felt mistreated. In their minds they accumulated trivial incidents in order to furnish proof for their accusations.

Individuals with PPD are difficult to get along with, and they often have problems with close relationships. Most of their relationships are filled with conflicts because they tend to always question the loyalties of others. Any deviation from 100 percent loyalty is interpreted as betrayal and will result in damaged relationships. Their lack of trust in others leads individuals with this disorder to fear intimacy, and when involved in intimate relationships, the partner usually has to prove his or her loyalty over and over again. As found in a study of jealousy, people with PPD seem to experience constant conflict with their spouses. Their excessive suspiciousness may be expressed in overt argumentativeness, in recurrent complaining, or by quiet, hostile aloofness. Their hypervigilance regarding potential threats and anticipated infidelity may lead them to act in a guarded, secretive, or devious manner or to subject the partner to frequent and lengthy interrogations. They often appear to be "cold" and lacking in tender feelings. They guard against loving and being loved. These distrustful and argumentative behaviors lead to dissolved partnerships and marriages ending in divorce (Dobbert, 2007).

Another description of paranoid personality points out that often, the presentation of conflict cases is made by a depressed, masochistic wife who can no longer tolerate the situation at home. In such cases, the husband usually has a paranoid personality and is resistant to treatment. The core of the personality organization in such cases is thought to consist of displacement of responsibility through projection, suspiciousness, defensive grandiosity, rigid conviction about one's beliefs, and concern over autonomy.

Up Close

Jennifer was driven by basic distrust and a need for perfection. On the surface, it seemed that she was happily married to Larry, who adored her, and doing a good job of raising their son. From Tom, her father, she had learned that one had to be vigilant about other people's motives—they were only too happy to betray others and take advantage of a trusting soul. Jennifer was constantly worried that other women would seduce Larry, who was not only good-looking but also successful in his career. Jennifer, who adhered to a strict diet, having only coffee and cigarettes for lunch, had no close female friends. Her interactions with females were restricted to superficial work-related exchanges in the doctor's office where she worked part-time and visits with her mother. Occasionally, Lisa, an attractive female cousin and her husband, would visit with Jennifer's family on some holidays. But Jennifer did not trust Lisa, either, and did not encourage the visits. Actually, Jennifer and Larry had met through Lisa, who worked for the same company as Larry did. Jennifer thought that Larry saw enough of her attractive cousin during the week at work. Having Lisa come to their house or visiting Lisa's home might amount to Larry having overexposure to Lisa.

Although Larry never gave her any reason to think that he was interested in having an affair with Lisa or any other woman, Jennifer could not control her suspicion, at times inquiring how often during the day he would meet Lisa at work. Jennifer could not relax and let go of her distrust because she knew from her father's teaching that people could not be trusted, and she also knew that even people as hyperalert about betrayal as her father could be fooled. After all, Jennifer knew how Harriett, her mother, had trained Tom to start his evening meal with a cup of coffee or two in order to remain ignorant of her shopping sprees. So in the end, whatever stories about betrayal and dishonesty Jennifer learned from her father found confirmation in her mother's behavior, who resorted to these relatively harmless schemes to make her own life with Tom and his paranoid personality disorder somewhat easier.

Theory and Research

Observations reported in the literature seem to indicate that subtle paranoid tendencies can be recognized in individuals from early childhood onward. These tendencies may gather further expressive coloration during adolescence before evolving into the full-blown picture of adult PPD. But further investigation will be needed (Conlon, 1984).

According to descriptive psychiatry literature, paranoid personality is genetically and phenomenologically related either to paranoia ("delusional disorder") or paranoid schizophrenia. The condition is characterized by the contradictory presence of (1) severe mistrust with naive gullibility,

(2) arrogant demandingness with hidden inferiority, (3) emotional coldness with marked sensitivity, (4) superficial asexuality with vulnerability to erotomania, (5) moralistic stance with potentially corrupt attitudes, and (6) extremely vigilant attention with inability to see the whole picture. This discrepancy between the outer persona and the inner world of the paranoid individual was noted by many authors and seemed to confirm the basic nature of the divided self of such a person (Akhtar, 1990).

During the 1980s, research efforts paid more attention to paranoid psychoses than to PPD. And when PPD was addressed, the focus usually remained on its potential relationship with paranoid schizophrenia or paranoid disorders but not on its phenomenological details. Even major reviews of personality literature paid little attention to the paranoid type, indicating that the condition has been understudied. For instance, a computer search of personality disorder literature from 1985 to 1988 yielded more than 1,200 citations, but not one was specifically addressing the phenomenology of PPD.

Experts emphasize the need to distinguish PPD from paranoid schizophrenia, reactive or acute paranoid disorders, and paranoia or "delusional disorder" (Akhtar, 1990). However, the psychiatric literature seems to indicate that PPD has a genetic and phenomenological relationship either to paranoia ("delusional disorder") or paranoid schizophrenia.

The line of demarcation between paranoia or "delusional disorder" and paranoid personality disorder is not easy to draw. The course of both disorders shows few changes; there are few exacerbations and few remissions. Intellectual and occupational functioning appear generally preserved in both disorders. In both disorders the content of paranoid complaints centers on marriage, plots, and being unfairly treated. The difference between paranoia and PPD seems to be one of a quantitative character (Stanton, 1978).

Some evidence indicates that a genetic contribution to paranoid traits and a possible genetic link between this personality disorder and schizophrenia exist. A large, long-term Norwegian study revealed PPD to be modestly heritable and to share a portion of its genetic and environmental risk factors with the other Cluster A personality disorders, schizoid and schizotypal (Kendler et al., 2006). A study investigating environmental influences found that adults who were subjected to verbal abuse in childhood were more than three times as likely to be diagnosed with paranoid or other (Cluster C) personality disorders as were adults who had no history of abuse. Abused or neglected children seem particularly vulnerable to paranoid and other personality disorders that reflect difficulties with trust, safety, and stability.

Other observations have led to suggestions of a subclassification within PPD. Authors proposed two subtypes: the first, a stronger, actively defiant, openly angry, and litigious type; and the second, a weaker, passive, secretive, and cynically brooding type. The former appears to have some similarities with narcissistic personality, whereas the latter seems to have a kinship with schizoid personality. While those linkages may make phenomenological and theoretical sense, it may also just be a matter of varying levels of social functioning manifested by individual patients rather than a matter of subtypes. Another explanation offered to account for the difference was the thought that the two paranoid styles are gender-related. The blatantly defiant picture may be more frequent among men, while the silently resentful outcome may be seen more often among women.

There has also been a focus of some theoretical considerations on the similarities and differences between PPD and obsessive-compulsive personality disorder, arguing that their similarities are as critical as their differences. Individuals with both disorders share a dislike for surprises and prefer order and predictability in their lives (Shapiro, 1965). However, unlike obsessive-compulsive individuals who know that the pressure to conform comes from within themselves, those with PPD view such demands as unjustified and coming from external sources. And they consciously plot against their imagined enemies. Compulsives rebel against their internalized moral authority in subtle, unconscious, and disguised ways, whereas paranoid individuals plot consciously against their imagined enemies (Fenichel, 1946).

On a cognitive level, compulsive individuals are overinclusive, but the paranoid individual's style is a narrowly focused, biased attention (Meissner, 1978). Where the compulsive individual is chronically indecisive and doubt-ridden, the paranoid is smugly self-assured. And on an interpersonal basis, compulsives are capable of concern and mutuality, but paranoid individuals view everyone with jealous mistrust (Volkan, 1976). There are also differences in the developmental backgrounds of the two conditions. Compulsives usually have had a successful separation-individuation process and have acquired self- and object constancy (Mahler, Pine, & Bergman, 1975), with problems arising from oedipal-phase difficulties that are regressively substituted by anal-phase metaphors. On the other hand, paranoid individuals had much actual pre-oedipal trauma, an unsuccessful separation-individuation, and a lack of self- and other-constancy (Akhtar & Byrne, 1983).

The many similarities between paranoid and narcissistic personality disorders make their distinction particularly difficult, and it may even be that cases with combined paranoid and narcissistic features are more common than their pure types (Millon, 1981).

Early descriptive psychiatrists have commented on the overlap between paranoid and antisocial personality disorders (Conlon, 1984). But although a developmental, psychostructural, and dynamic overlap may indeed exist between the two conditions, it is important to remember that individuals with PPD lack the chronicity of antisocial behavior (Reid, 1985).

The outcome of paranoid personality during middle and old age is perhaps better known. Studies of the presence of personality disorders in the elderly have suggested that paranoid individuals often make better adjustments to aging than their psychopathology would initially predict. Apparently, the fighting stance of paranoid personalities remains active insofar as failure is never their own. They have to singlehandedly continue their combat with the world at large, making life a diverting struggle against dangerous forces from the outside, leaving little time for despair and depression (Bergman, 1978).

Most authors have noted a discrepancy between the inner world of the person with paranoid personality disorder and his or her outer persona. As mentioned earlier, it seems that the condition is characterized by several contradictions, such as the coexistence of feelings of superiority and inferiority, the presence of profound mistrust with naive gullibility, hidden inferiority with arrogant demandingness, internal sensitivity with apparent emotional coldness, superficial asexuality with vulnerability to erotomania, and vigilant attention with inability to see the whole picture (Akhtar, 1990). It is thought that their fears may be counterbalanced by grandiose fantasies, obsessions with power and rank, and a simplistic, black-and-white view of the world (Bayer, 2000).

Attempting to synthesize developmental, dynamic, and descriptive features of PPD, some authors consider the discrepancy between the outer persona and the inner world of the afflicted person to be a more important feature than the usual focus on the classical triad of suspiciousness, feelings of persecution, and grandiosity. This frequently observed pervasive split involves the characteristics of self-concept, object relations, affects, morality, sexuality, and cognitive style. On the outside, paranoid individuals are arrogant, demanding, mistrustful, driven, moralistic, unromantic, and vigilant toward the surrounding environment. But internally they are frightened, timid, inconsiderate, self-doubting, gullible, vulnerable to erotomania, and unable to cognitively grasp the totality of events. It is argued that such a conceptualization would be beneficial because it combines descriptive and psychodynamic observations and correlates the behavioral and psychostructural (developmental) aspects of the paranoid personality pathology. In addition, it would provide help in diagnostically distinguishing paranoid from other related personality disorders.

Treatment

Treatment for paranoid personality disorder exists in the form of psychotherapy and medication. The prognosis for significant improvement depends on the person's commitment to lifelong treatment. Individuals who accept treatment can hold down jobs and maintain healthy relationships, but they must be willing to continue treatment throughout their lifetimes, because there is no cure for PPD. The symptoms of the disorder will continue but can be managed with care and support (Martel, 2017).

Treatment can be challenging because individuals with PPD have intense suspicion and mistrust of others, including psychotherapists. The trust to be established by the mental health professional should enable the patient to confide in the professional and believe and accept that they have a disorder. Often, people with PPD do not believe that their behavior is abnormal. To them it may seem completely rational to be suspicious of others.

Many individuals with PPD don't consider treatment. In general, people with personality disorders often do not seek out treatment until the disorder significantly interferes with their lives, which usually happens when their coping resources are stretched too thin to deal with stress or other life events (Bressert, 2017).

It has been observed that fewer than one in three adults with a personality disorder seek treatment. And although both psychotherapy and medication have been used in treating people with PPD, psychotherapy has not been very successful in most cases, mainly due to the significant distrust issue that is part of the condition. Treatment with antipsychotic medications such as risperidone or olanzapine, antidepressants, or antianxiety medication may be helpful for patients in overcoming some of the disorder's symptoms.

Other healthcare professionals discourage the use of medication for people with PPD because medications may contribute to a heightened sense of suspicion that can ultimately lead to the patient's withdrawal from therapy. However, for the treatment of specific conditions of the disorder, such as severe anxiety or delusions when these symptoms start to interfere with normal functioning, medications may be useful. In cases of severe anxiety or agitation, an antianxiety agent, such as diazepam, would be appropriate to prescribe. Antipsychotic medication—if the patient experiences severe agitation or delusional thinking—may be used for very brief intervals (Psychology Today, 2018).

Overall, most patients with this disorder experience symptoms for the duration of their lifetime and require consistent longtime, often intensive, therapy.

References

Akhtar, S. (1990). Paranoid personality disorder: A synthesis of developmental, dynamic, and descriptive features. *American Journal of Psychotherapy, 44*(1), 5–25.

Akhtar, S., & Byrne, J. P. (1983). The concept of splitting and its clinical relevance. *American Journal of Psychiatry, 140*, 1013–1016.

Bayer, L. (2000). *Personality disorders*. Philadelphia, PA: Chelsea House Publishers.

Beck, A. T., & Freeman, A. M. (1990). *Cognitive therapy of personality disorders*. New York, NY: Guilford Press.

Bergman, K. (1978). Neurosis and personality disorder in old age. In A. D. Issacs & F. Post (Eds.), *Studies in geriatric psychiatry* (pp. 41–76). New York, NY: John Wiley.

Bernstein, D. P., Useda, D., & Siever, L. J. (1995). Paranoid personality disorder. In J. W. Livesley (Ed.), *The DSM-IV personality disorders* (pp. 45–57). New York, NY: Guilford.

Bleuler, E. (1908). *Textbook of psychiatry* (Brill, A. A., Trans.). New York, NY: Macmillan Company, 1924.

Blum, H. (1981). Object inconsistency and paranoid conspiracy. *Journal of the American Psychoanalytical Association, 29*, 789–813.

Bressert, S. (2017). Paranoid personality disorder. *Psych Central*. Retrieved January 8, 2018, from https://psychcentral.com/disorders/paranoid-personality-disorder

Bursten, B. (1973). Some narcissistic personality types. *International Journal of Psychoanalysis, 54*, 287–290.

Cameron, N. (1963). *Personality development and psychopathology*. Boston, MA: Houghton Mifflin Company.

Conlon, G. B. (1984). The paranoid psychopath (Letter to the editor). *Medicine Journal, 97*, 90–91.

Dobbert, D. L. (2007). *Understanding personality disorders: An introduction*. Westport, CT: Praeger Publishers.

Erikson, E. H. (1950). *Childhood and society*. New York, NY: W. W. Norton.

Fenichel, O. (1946). *The psychoanalytic theory of neurosis*. New York, NY: W. W. Norton.

Freud, S. (1922). Some neurotic mechanisms in jealousy, paranoia and homosexuality. In *Standard edition* (Vol. 18, pp. 221–232). London: Hogarth Press.

Grant, B. F., Hasin, D. S., Simon, F. S., Dawson, D. A., Ruan, W. J., Goldstein, R. B., … Huang, B. (2004). Prevalence, correlates, and disability of personality disorders in the United States: Results from the National Epidemiologic Survey on Alcohol and related conditions. *Journal of Clinical Psychiatry, 65*(7), 948–958.

Hamilton, M. J. (1974). *Fish's clinical psychopathology*. Bristol: John Wright & Sons.

Healthy Place. (2016). What is paranoid personality disorder? Last updated July 20, 2016. Retrieved from https:www.healthyplace .com/personality-disorders/paranoid-personality-disorder/what-is -paranoid-personality-disorder

Heimann, P. (1952). Preliminary notes on some defense mechanisms in paranoid states. *International Journal of Psychoanalysis, 33*, 206–213.

Internet Mental Health—Paranoid personality disorder/2018 (http:// www.mentalhealth.com/dis/p20-pe01.html) Cited in WIKIPEDIA, retrieved 04/08/2018.

Jacobson, E. (1971). *Depression*. New York, NY: International Universities Press.

Jaspers, K. (1949). *General psychology* (J. Hoenig & M. Hamilton, Trans.). London: Manchester University Press, 1964.

Kendler, K. S., Czajkowski, N., Tambs, K., Torgersen, S., Aggen, S. H., Neale, M. C., & Reichborn-Kjennerud, T. (2006). Dimensional representations of DSM-IV cluster A personality disorders in a population-based sample of Norwegian twins: A multivariate study. *Psychological Medicine, 36*(11), 1583–1591.

Kernberg, O. F. (1975). *Borderline conditions and pathological narcissism*. New York, NY: Jason Aronson.

Klein, M. (1932). *The psychoanalysis of children* New York, NY: Norton & Co.

Kretschmer, E. (1927). *Der sensitive Beziehungswahn* (Vol. 2). Berlin: Springer.

Leonhard, K. (1959). *Die Aufteilung der Endogen Psychosen*. Berlin: Akademie.

Mahler, M., Pine, F., & Bergman, A. (1975). *The psychological birth of the human infant*. New York, NY: Basic Books.

Martel, J. (2017). Paranoid personality disorder. *Health Line*. Retrieved from https://www.healthline.com/health/paranoid-personality-disorder

Meissner, W. W. (1978). *The paranoid process*. New York, NY: Jason Aronson.

Millon, T. (1981). *Disorders of personality—DSM-III: Axis II*. New York, NY: John Wiley & Sons.

Polatin, P. (1975). Paranoid states. In A. M. Kaplan, H. I. Kaplan, & B. J. Sadock (Eds.), *Comprehensive textbook of psychiatry-II* (Vol. 1, pp. 992–1002). Baltimore: Williams & Wilkins.

Psychology Today. (2018). *Paranoid personality disorder*. Retrieved April 8, 2018, from https://www.psychologytoday.com/us/conditions/paranoid-personality-disorder

Reid, W. H. (1985). Antisocial personality. In R. Michels & J. O. Cavenar (Eds.), *Psychiatry* (Vol. 1, pp. 1–11, Section 1). Philadelphia, PA: Lippincott Co.

Salzman, L. (1974). Other character personality syndromes: Schizoid, inadequate, passive-aggressive, paranoid, dependent. In S. Ariety & E. B. Brody (Eds.), *American handbook of psychiatry* (2nd ed., Vol. 3). New York, NY: Basic Books.

Schneider, K. (1950). *Die psychopathischen Persönlichkeiten* [Psychopathic personalities]. Oxford, England: Franz Deuticke.

Shapiro, D. (1965). *Neurotic styles*. New York, NY: Basic Books.

Shepherd, M. (1961). Morbid jealousy: Some clinical and social aspects of psychiatric symptoms. *British Journal of Psychiatry, 107*, 687–714.

Slater, E., & Roth, M. (1977). *Clinical psychiatry*. London: Bailliere, Tindal.

Stanton, A. H. (1978). Personality disorders. In A. M. Nicholi (Ed.), *The Harvard guide to modern psychiatry*. Cambridge, MA: Belknap Press of Harvard University Press.

Volkan, V. D. (1976). *Primitive internalized object relations*. New York, NY: International Universities Press.

Winnicott, D. W. (1953). Psychosis and childcare. *British Journal of Medical Psychology, 26*(1), 68–74.

CHAPTER 9

Schizoid Personality Disorder

Symptoms, Diagnosis, and Incidence

The *DSM-5* lists as essential feature of schizoid personality disorder (SPD) a pervasive pattern of detachment from social relationships and a restricted range of emotional expressions in interpersonal settings. Beginning in early adulthood, this pattern can be observed in a variety of contexts. Individuals with SPD do not seem interested in developing close relationships or intimacy with others. Neither do they appear to derive satisfaction from being part of a family or other social group. They would rather spend time by themselves than with other people. Appearing socially isolated, they prefer solitary activities or hobbies to interacting with others. At times called "loners" by others, they prefer to involve themselves in mechanical tasks, computer or mathematical games, and abstract concepts, experiencing very little pleasure from sensory, bodily, or interpersonal experiences, such as walking on a beach at sunset or having sex. They usually do not have close friends or confidants.

Individuals with schizoid personality disorder appear not to be bothered by what others may think of them, and they seem indifferent to approval or criticism of others. They often do not respond appropriately to social cues and may be oblivious to the normal subtleties of social interaction. They rarely reciprocate gestures or facial expressions, such as smiles, displaying a "bland" exterior without visible emotional reactivity. According to their own reports, they rarely experience strong emotions and often display a constricted affect, appearing cold and aloof. They seem to have few goals and may just drift through life without definite directions. They usually don't date or marry.

In people with SPD, there seems to be a discrepancy between cognition and emotion that characterizes all aspects of their mental life, leading to a concomitant uncertainty about their experiences and to an impoverished self-concept. As a result, many of these individuals fail to develop a coherent sense of direction and purpose in life. They show an insensitivity to social norms and conventions.

Although SPD is not the same as schizophrenia or schizotypal personality disorder, some evidence exists of links and shared genetic risk between SPD, other Cluster A personality disorders, and schizophrenia. Therefore, SPD is considered to be a "schizophrenia-like personality disorder" (Esterberg, 2010).

Another running theme for people with SPD is suicide, although they are not likely to actually attempt it. The idea of suicide functions like a driving force against the person's schizoid defenses (Masterson & Klein, 1995).

It has been argued that the definition of SPD is flawed due to cultural bias. Furthermore, it has been suggested that SPD does not constitute a mental disorder but is simply an avoidant attachment style that requires more distant emotional proximity (Panagiotis, 2012). If this is true, many of the problematic reactions exhibited by these individuals in social situations may be partly accounted for by the judgments commonly imposed on people with these characteristics.

Under stress, some individuals with SPD features may occasionally experience brief episodes of reactive psychosis. In terms of comorbidity, the personality disorders that most frequently co-occur are schizotypal, paranoid, and avoidant personality disorders (Ekleberry, 2008). Alexithymia, the inability to identify and describe emotions, seems to have a strong relationship with SPD, but they do not constitute the same condition (Coolidge, 2012).

The substitution of a nonhuman object for a human object is a defense action of people with SPD, which often establishes a trace of a personal feeling about the relationship. According to the object relations view, drug use and alcoholism reinforce the fantasy of linkage with an internal object while enabling the addict to be indifferent to the external object world, which makes addiction a schizoid and symbiotic defense (Seinfeld, 1991).

The single most egosyntonic drug for individuals with SPD may be marijuana because it permits a detached state of fantasy and distance from others. It also provides a richer internal experience than these individuals can normally create for themselves, and it reduces an internal sense of emptiness and failure to participate in life. In addition, readily available and safe to obtain, alcohol is another obvious drug of choice for these individuals. People are likely to use these substances in isolation for the effect on internal processes (Ekleberry, 2008).

In clinical settings, schizoid personality disorder is uncommon. An estimate based on a probability subsample from Part II of the National Comorbidity Survey Replication mentions a prevalence of 4.9 percent, while data from the 2001–2002 National Epidemiologic Survey on Alcohol and Related Conditions suggests a 3.1 percent prevalence of schizoid personality disorder. It is diagnosed slightly more often in males and may cause more impairment in them. Overall, this personality disorder is rare.

Timeline

1908   Eugen Bleuler coined the word *schizoid*.

1910   August Hoch introduced a similar concept, the "shut-in" personality.

1925   Ernst Kretschmer coined the term *schizothyme* for former schizoid people.

1926   Early account of "schizoid psychopathology" provided by Russian psychiatrist Dr. Grunya Sukhareva about a group of children resembling today's SPD and Aspergers.

1933   Pyotr Gannushkin also included *Schizoids* and *Dreamers* in his detailed typology of personality types.

1940   Ronald Fairbairn presented seminal work on the schizoid personality, describing "schizoid exhibitionism," among other characteristics.

2013   Psychiatrist Salman Akhtar provided a clinical case study of a schizoid man as an illustration of his phenomenological profile.

History

The prefix *schizo* derives from the Greek word meaning "split," but neither schizophrenia nor schizoid (or schizotypal) personality disorder refer to what is commonly called a split personality.

Eugen Bleuler used the term *schizoid* to designate a human tendency to direct attention toward one's inner life, away from the external world. The concept is akin to introversion in that it was not thought of in terms of psychopathology. Bleuler called the exaggeration of this tendency the "schizoid personality" (Akhtar, 1987). His description of these personalities was that they are "comfortably dull and at the same time sensitive, people who in a narrow manner pursue vague purposes"; and similarly, characteristics of Hoch's "shut-in" personality included among others reticence, reclusiveness, shyness, and a preference for living in a fantasy world (Livesley & West, 1986).

Emil Kraepelin (1919), the father of present-day psychiatry, mentioned childhood precursors of some types of schizophrenia, such as a quiet, shy, and retiring disposition, especially in boys. Girls seemed to show sensitiveness, excitability, irritability, and self-willedness (Wolff, 1995).

The Swiss psychiatrist Eugen Bleuler described people who were shut-in, suspicious, sensitive, comfortably dull, and pursuing vague purposes as "schizoid."

Ernst Kretschmer (1925) described schizoid or "schizothyme" people, as he called them, as being unsociable, oversensitive, stubborn, pedantic, and also cold and lacking in "affective resonance." "A certain unreasonableness" and inaccessibility to argument, with preconceived notions and superstitions, were characteristics included by others. It was thought that some schizoid individuals may turn to vegetarianism and fanatical outdoor activities and become people who shut their ears to reason, becoming completely absorbed in some idea (Essen-Moeller, 1946).

A report published in 1926 is perhaps the first account of schizoid children. The report consisted of six case studies at the hospital school of the Moscow psychoneurological children's inpatient department. The six boys ranged in age from 2 to 14 years and had been unlike other children since early childhood. They were solitary, excessively sensitive, yet superficial in their responses to others. Five of the boys were of above average intelligence, several came from gifted families, and their parents seemed to have similar traits. The Russian psychiatrist Dr. Grunya Sukhareva's diagnosis of these children was "schizoid personality disorder of childhood," thinking they were like Kretschmer's schizoid types in that they had an inborn predisposition to an unusual personality. While these cases shared some characteristics of schizophrenia, their course was different from that of schizophrenia patients; they showed no deterioration as they grew older (Wolff, 1995).

Kraepelin and others noticed some similarity between the features of SPD and the symptoms of schizophrenia. They confirmed the high prevalence of schizoid personality in the past histories of schizophrenic patients and in their biological relatives.

Originally, the concept of the schizoid character, as developed by Ernst Kretschmer, consisted of an amalgamation of avoidant, schizotypal, and schizoid traits. Finally, in 1980, with the work of Theodore Millon, the schizoid character was split into three personality disorders—what are now schizoid, schizotypal, and avoidant personality disorders. Since then the debate has been ongoing about whether that is accurate or if perhaps these traits are different expressions of the same personality disorder (Livesley & West, 1986).

It was Theodore Millon who restricted the term *schizoid* to only those personalities who are lacking the capacity to establish social relationships with others, characterizing their way of thinking as being vague and empty and of at times having impaired perceptual scanning. This may be the reason for some people with SPD to miss the fine details of life (Beck & Freeman, 1990). In Millon's opinion, SPD is different from other personality disorders because it is the personality disorder without a personality. This may be due to the current diagnostic criteria as they describe SPD only in terms of an absence of certain traits, which results in a "deficit syndrome" or a "vacuum." The fact that the criteria mention only what is lacking, instead of delineating the presence of something, makes it difficult to describe and to research such a concept (Millon, 2004).

The architects of *DSM-III* attempted to subdivide and sharpen the boundaries of its heterogeneous diagnosis of SPD by adding schizotypal and paranoid personality disorders to the "odd" cluster and moving avoidant personality disorder to the "anxious" cluster, which resulted in a narrowing of the SPD diagnosis, raising additional questions about its diagnostic boundaries and about whether the diagnosis is a valid separate entity (Mittal, Kalus, Bernstein, & Siever, 2007).

There has also been another suggestion that two different disorders would give a better representation of SPD. One of these would be an affect-constricted disorder (belonging to schizotypal personality disorder) and the other being a seclusive disorder (belonging to avoidant personality disorder). Other voices have called for the removal of the SPD category from future editions of the *DSM* and replacing it with a dimensional model (Skodol, 2011).

In the more recent diagnostic classifications, the meaning of *schizoid personality disorder* has become more restricted, and a new category, schizotypal personality disorder, has been formed for personality characteristics previously subsumed under the term *schizoid*.

Of interest to note is that the *DSM-5* classification schizoid personality disorder lists seven diagnostic criteria, whereas the Classification of

Mental and Behavioural Disorders of *ICD-10* lists nine diagnostic criteria. Nine criteria of the schizoid personality were also suggested by Harry Guntrip, with one of them being narcissism (Masterson & Klein, 1995, pp. 13–23). The description of Guntrip's nine characteristics would clarify some differences between the traditional *DSM* profile of SPD and the traditional informed object relations view (Masterson & Klein, 1995).

Development and Causes

There are many theories regarding the possible causes for SPD, and most professionals subscribe to a biopsychosocial model of causation.

SPD is more likely to be observed in people whose relatives have schizophrenia or SPD. As suggested by some evidence, there are shared genetic and environmental risk factors among the Cluster A personality disorders, and there is an increased occurrence of SPD in relatives of people with schizophrenia and schizotypal personality disorder (Esterberg, 2010).

As suggested by the findings of twin studies with SPD traits, such as low sociability and low warmth, these traits seem to be inherited. Heritability estimates of SPD range from 50 percent to 59 percent (Blaney, 2014). Other research and clinical work with children and teenagers with schizoid symptoms have indicated a constitutional—probably genetic—basis in schizoid personality (Wolff, 1995). Additionally, the involvement of biological factors may be indicated by the link between SPD and being underweight (Mather, 2008). Other risk factors for being afflicted with mental disorders and contributing to the development of schizoid personality disorder include prenatal caloric malnutrition, premature birth, and low birth weight. And those individuals who have experienced traumatic brain injury may also be at risk of developing schizoid-like personality traits (Abel, 2010; Martens, 2010; Brigham Young University, 2014).

The solitariness, poor relationships, and underachievement in school that mark individuals with SPD may first be noticeable in childhood and adolescence, emphasizing their difference and making them subject to teasing.

Effects and Costs

Social consequences of inappropriate responses, family disruptions, loss of employment and housing—all are sometimes the costs of suffering from schizoid personality disorder.

Schizoid individuals' lack of desire to be in a close relationship or even be part of a family usually results in an impoverished emotional life. Furthermore, as they also do not take pleasure in many activities, their lives may be less productive than would seem normal and healthy.

Because of their lack of meaningful communication with other people, those who are diagnosed with SPD are unable to develop accurate impressions of how well they get along with others. As they are challenged to achieve self-awareness of the impact of their own actions in social situations, their self-image becomes empty, making them feel unreal (Laing, 1965).

A significant part of the schizoid person's withdrawal from the world is a pathological reliance on fantasizing, combined with a preoccupation with inner experiences. In this way, fantasy becomes a core component of the "self in exile"—a complicated process that facilitates the individual's withdrawal (Masterson & Klein, 1995). Fantasy can be viewed as a relationship with the world and with others by proxy. Being a substitute relationship, it is characterized by idealized, defensive and compensatory mechanisms. This fantasy system, or substitute relationship, is self-contained within the individual and free from the dangers and anxieties normally associated with emotional connections to real people and situations. The fantasy permits schizoid individuals to feel connected (to internal objects), but still free from the imprisonment in relationships (Masterson & Klein, 1995; Laing, 1965; Winnicott, 2012).

Schizoid people's preference to remain alone and detached may cause their need for sex to be less than that of those who do not suffer from SPD. They sometimes appear sexually apathetic; although they do not typically suffer from anorgasmia, they may feel that their personal space is violated with sexual activities. Masturbation or sexual abstinence appears preferable to the emotional closeness they would have to tolerate when having sex (Nannarello, 1953).

Although individuals with SPD appear to prefer leading a solitary existence with solitary activities, there may be a high price to pay for this preference. As research has shown, social isolation and loneliness may pose greater public health hazards than obesity, and they significantly increase the risk for premature mortality (Wood, 2017).

Due to their lack of interest in social relationships, individuals with SPD who lack financial resources may be at a greater risk for homelessness than other people without this disorder (Rouff, 2000). Actually, there is a high rate of SPD and other Cluster A personality disorders (up to 92%) among homeless people (Connolly, 2008).

It has been speculated that schizoid personality disorder may have links to creativity as observed in a study including two samples of college students (n = 40 each) drawn from a larger sample (N = 188). The students were identified as either high creative or low creative, based on their performance on five measures of creativity. Following their performances they participated in a videotaped semi-structured interview. The video recordings were assessed as to the utilization of 15 ego defense styles. Thirteen of the 15 ego defense styles showed statistically significant mean differences, with high creatives scoring higher on schizoid characteristics (Domino et al., 2002).

In Society

People with SPD rarely function as interactive parts of society. They are not interested in seeking social contacts. Rarely are they concerned about receiving either approval or criticism from others (Rasmussen, 2005).

Due to their withdrawn, self-absorbed, and socially inept behaviors, their existence can be understood to occur only at the periphery of society. Their detachment and general lack of reciprocity with gestures, smiles, or facial expressions tend to characterize social interaction and communication as awkward, uncomfortable, and strange. As people in general expect others to express some opinions and emotions, the person with SPD, in his or her indifference to others' thoughts and feelings, appears to be a member of a different and unknown culture, like someone from outer space.

The lack of social and emotional responsiveness of individuals with SPD is often irritating to others, who then tend to being even more intrusive, demanding a response. This is an important aspect in therapy sessions because it may lead to the patient's further withdrawal from the therapist.

Underlying the lack of responsiveness is a fear of closeness. People with this disorder perceive others as intrusive. Their boundary problems occur as feelings of vulnerability in interpersonal encounters. Their response is to withdraw into a "shell" of their own making.

Lack of responsiveness or restricted expression go hand-in-hand with intimacy problems. As emotions establish bonds, it is difficult to be close to someone who does not express feelings. Therefore, the schizoid person's reluctance to exhibit emotions ensures that nobody will come close enough—emotionally and mentally—to really get to know the schizoid person. Many people with SPD are also secretive because they feel vulnerable and exposed when any information about them is revealed to others (Fairbairn, 1952). They may go so far as to refuse to introduce close relatives or friends to other people they know for fear that these relatives will be sources of information about the schizoid person. Also, the impression those relatives would make on others might give them details about the schizoid individual for which they could judge or criticize the schizoid person.

Schizoid individuals may have particular difficulty expressing anger, even when they are directly provoked. They often react passively to adverse circumstances and have trouble responding appropriately to important life events. This often gives others the impression that the schizoid person lacks emotion. Often their lives seem to be without direction, and they may appear to drift in their goals.

It is possible for people with SPD to form relationships with others based on intellectual, physical, occupational, or recreational activities as long as there is no need or request for emotional intimacy, because schizoid individuals "prefer to make relationships on their own terms and not in terms of the impulses of other people." If they cannot attain that, they prefer isolation (Winnicott, 2008, p. 73).

Up Close

Marianne, a single woman in her late 20s, had always been a solitary person, which at times she camouflaged by participating in team activities, although she was never a real member of the team. It was just one of the many activities and interests she pursued but never carried to completion. This tendency characterized most of Marianne's life. Whenever she embarked upon a new interest, her mother would ask her, "Are you going to finish this one for a change?" Her mother's question did not lead Marianne to change except for trying not to tell her mother about any further endeavors. This became easier when Marianne moved into her own apartment in another town about 250 miles from home where she had found employment as a clerk in a bank. She did not mind the superficial contact with customers and coworkers but stayed away from any more meaningful relationships. Her dating history played out on an equally superficial basis.

However, underneath this seemingly uneventful facade, Marianne developed a secret life. Though she found any prolonged romantic relationship too intrusive and restrictive, she felt an urge and curiosity about sex. From time to time Marianne by herself ventured out into one of the town's bars. The clothes she wore on these outings were quite different in style and colors from those she wore to work or other regular activities. She used similar differences in her hairstyles and makeup, creating something like two different versions of herself.

It usually did not take long after entering the bar for Marianne to find a man inviting her to a drink or two, including spending the evening.

Marianne never took any of the men to her place; all the sexual encoun-ters took place either in the man's home or in a hotel. Although Mari-anne was certainly intelligent enough to understand the risks she faced engaging in the activities of her secret life, the confrontation with emo-tional openness and disclosure of her innermost personality that would be expected in a normal romantic relationship were too disturbing to even consider. As might be expected, after some time, Marianne had to admit to herself that one of the risks had caught up with her: she had contracted a sexually transmitted disease.

At Work

Among the list of symptoms that characterize this disorder, the individu-al's preference for solitary activities, enjoyment of few activities, indiffer-ence to praise or criticism, and emotional detachment are the ones that will most likely interfere with the development of mutually satisfying work relationships.

Occupationally, people with SPD are impaired in work situations because of their inability to interact with coworkers. Most of them are unable to participate in friendly banter with colleagues or otherwise cooperate in team efforts (Bayer, 2000). Therefore, they would be more appropriately placed with computer work or individually performed mechanical tasks, except for their lack of goal-directedness, which may require more intense supervision than is usual in most workplaces.

As schizoid individuals tend to hide their emotions, presumably to avoid social contact and being known by others, many of them are at the same time hypersensitive. If these inhibited individuals experience dis-comfort in intrusive relationships, their reaction is withdrawal—actual social withdrawal or creation of a facade behind which to hide the real self. As the need for hiding or withdrawal increases, the individual finds it more and more difficult to access his or her real self, which bestows a lack of authenticity upon the individual's experiences (Livesley, 2003). This, in turn, may lead to difficulties with self-direction. Nothing seems worth pursuing; tentative goals fall by the wayside if they are presenting any hurdles. A general passivity creates problems with the schizoid indi-vidual's ability to accomplish or complete tasks, not only in the personal life sphere but even more so in work situations.

In addition, their indifference to criticism or approval may prevent the development of a mutually successful work setting because supervisors and coworkers are left without tools to regulate or improve the schizoid individual's productivity if interpersonal communication is required.

Up Close

It was six days before his 33rd birthday when Noah lost his job—again. It was his second job loss this year, and there had been several in years past. It wasn't that Noah was not intelligent enough to perform his job duties as a truck driver making deliveries for a local company. And he had no difficulty interacting with others on a superficial level. Noah was a reliable employee, always on time to start the day's deliveries—as long as everything went according to schedule. Problems arose when sudden changes in the schedule or the locations for deliveries required Noah to make decisions about how best to handle those changes. Debating within himself on how to accommodate the required changes, Noah felt stressed out and unable to make a decision. Often he told himself that he needed to rest his mind before deciding on any new approach, and, almost as often, he wasted enough time with his indecision that in the end the deliveries were late or, even worse, impossible to carry out because there was nobody left to receive or accept them at their points of destination. The frequency of sudden changes in established routines was not high, but the consequences of Noah's prolonged decision process made them quite noticeable.

Now Noah was confronted with the need to call Susan, his ex-wife, and explain why his child support payment was going to be late again.

It had been a brief marriage. Susan and Noah had met in their church group as both had volunteered time to help with some of the community events that the church sponsored. Susan had felt comfortable with Noah because he seemed to respect her personal space, never coming too close (physically or emotionally) to her during any of their interactions. Their dating activities occurred mostly in connection with some church events. Noah appeared respectful and protective of Susan's state of virginity and refrained from initiating sexual advances. After their wedding they had sex a few times, but Noah did not seem interested or appear to derive much pleasure from it. But it was enough to get Susan pregnant. After the birth of their little daughter, sexual activity did not become more frequent, and Susan, feeling unloved, finally left Noah.

Noah felt sadness over the loss of his family, but even the sadness did not feel like his own. It was more like he observed some other person going through the end of a marriage.

In Relationships

Individuals with SPD don't seem to derive any pleasure from being part of a family or other social group and refrain as much as possible from any social participation. They seem to experience acute discomfort in close relationships. Being oblivious to the interests, emotions, and opinions of others, schizoid individuals appear cold and aloof, rarely expressing feelings like joy or anger. As they remain strangers to those around them, intimacy cannot develop. Furthermore, the low interest in sexual activities and the reduced pleasure experienced from sensory, bodily, or erotic activity induces the schizoid individual to avoid intimacy or even the presence of others and engage in solitary activities or hobbies instead.

Restricted expression is consistent with intimacy problems experienced by people with SPD; many of them are secretive because they feel exposed and vulnerable if they reveal information about themselves. They usually are excessively self-reliant and avoid care- or help-seeking behavior because it requires contact with other people.

Individuals with SPD exhibit oversensitivity regarding their own ideas and feelings while at the same time being insensitive to the feelings of others. This combination does not contribute to harmonious relationships. Due to their lack of social skills and their lack of desire for intimacy and for sexual experiences, individuals with SPD have few friendships, date infrequently, and often do not marry (Bressert, 2017).

Up Close
By their eighth wedding anniversary, Ralph had learned the procedures that would get him through the event: loading flowers, chocolate, and a bottle of wine into his shopping cart at the local supermarket and making reservations for an early dinner at their favorite restaurant that featured a huge food buffet. It had to be an early dinner because Ralph worked nights, servicing the computer systems at a hospital chain. Sometimes he had to travel during the day to another part of the state where one of the hospitals was located. What Ralph liked best about his job was that he was not required to interact much with people. Early in his life, in high school, he developed an interest in computers. The computer understood him—not like in school, when he had asked the teacher a question about something he didn't understand. The teacher acted like he did not understand Ralph's question, and some of his classmates snickered. Ralph never asked again. He didn't make or seem to need any friends. His grades in high school were mediocre, except for mathematics, which he liked. After graduation from high school, he managed to get into the community college and embarked upon a career in information technology. He never dated and did not seem interested in a sexual relationship—at least not with another person. Secretly, he indulged in watching pornography and masturbating. The idea of sharing the intimacy of his thoughts and body with anyone scared him.

After the completion of his training, he obtained the job he was still working at. Working night shifts was not only convenient because of the minimal interactions he had to face with others, it also came in handy when he married Julie, a distant cousin who had come to visit with his parents. And she stayed long enough to get herself a job as a bookkeeper at one of the local banks.

As Ralph found out later, the reason for Julie's visit had been that her father had sexually abused her for several years, and Ralph's parents agreed to have Julie live with them so she would be removed from the unhealthy situation without many people knowing the reason behind it. Probably as a result of the years of sexual abuse, Julie did not experience any desire for sex, and she hated to have her body touched.

Ralph and Julie seemed to be made for each other. It was a safe marriage. Except for weekends, Ralph and Julie spent only a couple of hours together, since she worked during the day and Ralph spent most nights at his job. During the day, when he had the home to himself, he could indulge in watching pornography without becoming anxious about Julie's presence. On special occasions, such as their anniversary, they could squeeze in a short early dinner for celebration.

Ralph's parents were somewhat disappointed when over the years there was no sign of grandchildren.

Theory and Research

In an early study of 500 consecutive child-guidance clinic attendees, 75 were labeled as "schizoid," reflecting a schizoid cluster comprising characteristics such as fantastic thinking, daydreaming, lack of concentration, carelessness, and regression toward infantile behavior. But these children came from socioeconomically superior families and had no adverse background factors to account for their difficulties (Jenkins & Glickman, 1946).

Comparing personality disorders and Myers-Briggs Type Indicator types in a University of Colorado Springs (2001) study, it was found that SPD had a significant correlation with the Introverted (I) and Thinking (T) preferences.

According to the AARP Loneliness Study, there is evidence that social isolation and loneliness increase the risk for premature mortality. The study involved data from two meta-analyses. The first involved 148 studies, representing more than 300,000 participants, and revealed that greater social connection is associated with a 50 percent reduced risk for premature mortality. The second meta-analysis included 70 studies with more than 3.4 million participants primarily from North America but also from Europe, Asia, and Australia. The focus was on the role that factors such as social isolation, loneliness, or living alone might have on mortality. It was found that all three factors had equal and significant effects on the risk of premature death—effects that were equal to or exceeded the effects of other well-accepted risk factors (Wood, 2017).

Research has shown that there appears to be a strong link between schizoid personality disorder and the development of other problems, such as schizophrenia (Rodriguez & DeChavez, 2000) and homelessness (Rouff, 2000). Similarly, observations of depressed patients undergoing a 6-month treatment with fluoxetine revealed that the presence of symptoms of schizoid personality disorder was associated with poorer outcome of treatment (Mulder, Joyce, Frampton, Luty, & Sullivan, 2006).

A study investigating the possibility of a specific link between Cluster A comorbidity and increased stress appraisal in depressed patients indicated that the persistent pattern of detachment from social relationships resulting in emotional coldness so characteristic of schizoid personality disorder might be the connection (Candrian et al., 2008).

Studies on the schizoid personality have developed along two different paths: the "descriptive psychiatry" tradition, which focuses on overtly observable behavioral and describable symptoms (with its clearest exposition in the *DSM-5*), and the "dynamic psychiatry" tradition, which includes the exploration of covert or unconscious motivations and character structure as elaborated by classic psychoanalysts and object-relations theory.

The descriptive tradition had its start with Ernst Kretschmer's description of observable schizoid behaviors, which organized into three groups of characteristics (Kretschmer, 1931):

1. unsociability, quietness, reservedness, seriousness, eccentricity,
2. timidity, shyness with feelings, sensitivity, nervousness, excitability, fondness of nature and books,
3. pliability, kindliness, honesty, indifference, silence, cold emotional attitudes.

These characteristics were the precursors of the *DSM-III* partitioning of the schizoid character into three distinct personality disorders: schizotypal, avoidant, and schizoid. However, Kretschmer did not intend to divide these behaviors into isolated characteristics but rather conceived of them as being simultaneously present as varying potentials in schizoid individuals. In Kretschmer's opinion, the majority of schizoids are not *either* oversensitive *or* cold, but they are oversensitive and cold "at the same time" in different relative proportions, tending to move along these dimensions from one behavior to the other (Kretschmer, 1931).

The second path, that of dynamic psychiatry, started with observations by Eugen Bleuler (1924), who observed that the schizoid person and schizoid pathology were not different entities (Masterson & Klein, 1995). Then Fairbairn delineated four central schizoid themes:

1. the need to regulate interpersonal distance as a central focus of concern,
2. the ability to mobilize self-reliance and self-preservative defenses,
3. a pervasive tension between the anxiety-laden need for attachment and the defensive need for distance that is expressed in observable behavior as *indifference*, and
4. an overvaluation of the inner world at the expense of the outer world.

Following Fairbairn, the dynamic psychiatry tradition has continued to explore the schizoid character.

Withdrawal or detachment from others, a characteristic feature of schizoid pathology, apparently may appear either in "classic" or "secret" form. In the classic form, it matches the typical description of the schizoid personality as described in the *DSM-5*. But just as often, it may be a hidden internal state. In other words, what appears on the surface, the objective observation, may not match the internal subjective world of the schizoid individual. As early as 1940, Fairbairn recognized and described the phenomenon of "schizoid exhibitionism," in which the schizoid individual can express feeling and can make what appear to be impressive social contacts but, in reality, gives nothing and loses nothing because he or she is playing a part. The real personality remains uninvolved below the surface. According to Fairbairn, *the person* disowns the part that is played by him or her while the schizoid individual seeks to preserve his or her personality intact and free from compromise (Fairbairn, 1952). Some researchers have given descriptions of SPD individuals who would apparently "enjoy" public speaking engagements but experienced great difficulty during breaks when the audience members would attempt to engage them emotionally (Seinfeld, 1991).

The sometimes sexually apathetic behavior of individuals with SPD—while not leading to systematic research efforts—has aroused theoretical thinking attempting to explain the phenomenon. It has been described how some married schizoid individuals may embark upon "secret sexual affairs" as attempts to reduce the quantity of emotional intimacy within a single relationship (Guntrip, 1969). As pointed out by Karen Horney (1999), the schizoid person's sexual resignation carries the appeal of freedom; sex may be excluded from a permanent relationship because it feels too intimate, but instead, the person's sexual needs are satisfied with a stranger. On the other hand, the individual may restrict a relationship to only sexual activities without sharing other experiences with the partner (Horney, 1999). As an example of what Jeffrey Seinfeld (1991) called "schizoid hunger," behaviors that actually reflect sexual promiscuity may be used by a schizoid woman secretly visiting bars to meet men for the purpose of obtaining impersonal sexual gratification, which seem to alleviate her feelings of hunger and emptiness, as described in the Up Close vignette "In Society."

Contrary to the proposition that schizoid individuals are either sexual or asexual, other suggestions indicated that *both* these forces may be present in individuals, despite their rather opposite aims (Akhtar, 1987).

Based on a clinical case study of a schizoid man, psychiatrist Salman Akhtar developed a phenomenological profile of SPD in which classic and contemporary views are synthesized with psychoanalytic observations. The clinical features of the profile involve six areas of psychosocial functioning, which are organized by "overt" and "covert" manifestations. The meanings of "overt" and "covert" here do not classify them as different subtypes but as traits that may occur simultaneously within one single individual. These designations do not suggest that they are conscious or unconscious, but they denote seemingly contradictory aspects that are phenomenologically easily discernable. This method of organizing symptomatology emphasizes the centrality of splitting and identity confusion in SPD (Akhtar, 1987).

A clinically accurate picture of schizoid sexuality is expected to include the overt signs of asexuality, occasional celibacy, absence of romantic interests, and aversion to sexual gossip and innuendo, as well as covert manifestations, such as secret voyeuristic and pornographic interests, vulnerability to erotomania, and a tendency toward perversion. However, none of these characteristics necessarily applies to all people with SPD.

Upon reviewing information from relevant publications and from databases of personality disorders study groups regarding psychometric characteristics of SPD, it was noted that comparatively little evidence exists for the validity and reliability of SPD as a separate, multifaceted personality disorder. There was some contention that the group of patients termed "schizoid" actually represented two distinct groups, an "affect constricted" group, who might fit better within schizotypal personality disorder, and a "seclusive" group, who might better be subsumed within avoidant personality disorder. The research-based justification for retaining SPD as an independent diagnosis is sparse (Triebwasser, Chemerinski, Roussos, & Siever, 2012).

Other researchers also have voiced concerns about distinguishing schizoid personality disorder from other phenomenologically similar personality disorders in Cluster A and from avoidant personality disorder (Mittal et al., 2007). Additional investigations are needed to determine whether SPD is part of the schizophrenia spectrum. Further research should incorporate biological markers (e.g., deviant smooth eye tracking, attention deficits) that have been observed in schizotypal personality disorder and schizophrenia.

Treatment

Not much research has been done regarding the treatment of schizoid personality disorder, partly because individuals with this diagnosis typically do not experience their social isolation as a problem, and they don't compete with or envy people who enjoy close relationships.

An individual therapy plan that can establish a long-term level of trust may be of benefit in some cases of SPD by providing patients with an outlet for transforming their false perceptions of friendships into authentic relationships. Very gradually, individual psychotherapy may bring about the formation of a true relationship between the patient and therapist. However, in general, long-term psychotherapy is not recommended because of its poor treatment outcomes and the costs inherent in lengthy therapy. Instead, it is recommended that therapy focus on simple treatment goals to alleviate current troubling concerns or stressors within the individual's life. Cognitive restructuring may be a way to address some types of clear, irrational thoughts that are influencing the patient's behaviors in negative ways. However, it is important to clearly define the therapeutic plan at the onset of treatment. Group therapy, generally a potentially effective treatment modality, is not considered to be a good initial treatment, because at first, patients would tend to withdraw from the group. But if they were to remain, they might grow participatory as the level of discomfort gradually decreases (Psychology Today, 2017). Another vehicle for treatment might be in the form of socialization groups and educational strategies in which people with SPD identify their positive and negative emotions. Such identifiers could help individuals to learn about their own emotions and the emotions they elicit from others and to experience the common emotions with other people with whom they relate on some basis.

Yet another source suggests that treatment of SPD typically involves long-term psychotherapy with an experienced therapist, and prescription of medication may help with specific troubling and debilitating symptoms (Bressert, 2017). There has been some concern that for the most part, psychotherapy alone has not been effective with this condition. Thus, in some instances, medication can be beneficial in bringing some symptoms under control, so psychotherapy can assist the individual in his or her daily life.

The schizoid patient may not have many symptoms that can be addressed with medication. But antianxiety drugs may be of some help in dealing with the tension they often experience. Additionally, low-dose antipsychotics may reduce distorted thoughts and depression. A careful choice of medication may be helpful in having patients function well in the everyday world. Over the past several decades, drug therapy has been helpful in reducing hospital stays for the disorder. But overall, SPD is very rare in clinical settings; most physicians seldom come across it (Bayer, 2000).

Because SPD is a poorly studied disorder with little clinical data available, the effectiveness of psychotherapeutic and pharmacological treatments for the disorder have yet to be empirically and systematically investigated (MedlinePlus, 2014).

References

Abel, K. M. (2010). Birth weight, schizophrenia and adult mental disorder: Is risk confined to the smallest babies? *Archives of General Psychiatry, 67*(9), 923–930.

Akhtar, S. (1987). Schizoid personality disorder: A synthesis of developmental, dynamic, and descriptive features. *American Journal of Psychotherapy, 41*(4), 400–518.

Bayer, L. (2000). *Personality disorders.* Philadelphia, PA: Chelsea House Publishers.

Beck, A. T., & Freeman, A. (1990). *Cognitive therapy of personality disorders* (1st ed., p. 125). New York, NY: The Guilford Press.

Blaney, P. H. (2014). *Oxford textbook of psychopathology.* New York, NY: Oxford University Press.

Bleuler, E. (1924). *Textbook of psychiatry.* New York, NY: Macmillan.

Bressert, S. (2017). Schizoid personality disorder. *Psych Central.* Retrieved December 26, 2017, from https://psychcentral.com/disorders/schizoid-personality-disorder/

Brigham Young University. (2014). Right frontal pole cortical thickness and social competence in children with chronic traumatic brain injury. *Journal of Head Trauma Rehabilitation, 30*, E24–E31.

Candrian, M., Schwartz, F., Farabaugh, A., Perlis, R. H., Ehlert, U., & Fava, M. (2008) Personality disorders and perceived stress in Major Depressive Disorder. *Psychiatry Research, 160*(2), 184–191.

Connolly, A. J. (2008). Personality disorders in homeless drop-in center clients. *Journal of Personality Disorders, 22*(6), 573–588.

Coolidge, F. L. (2012). Are alexithymia and schizoid personality disorder synonymous diagnoses? *Comprehensive Psychiatry, 54*(2), 141–148.

Coolidge, F. L., Segal, D. L., Hook, J. N., Yamazaki, T. G., & Ellett, J. A. C. (2001). An empirical investigation of Jung's personality types and psychological disorder features. *Journal of Psychological Type, 58*, 33–36. Retrieved August 10, 2013, from http://www.uccs.edu/Documents/dsegal/An-empirical-investigation-Jungs-types-and-PD-features-JPT-2.pdf

Domino, G., Short, J., Evans, A., & Romano, P. (2002). Creativity and ego defense mechanisms: Some exploratory empirical evidence. *Creativity Research Journal, 14*(1), 17–25.

Ekleberry, S. C. (2008). *Integrated treatment for co-occurring disorders: Personality disorders and addiction* (pp. 31–32). New York, NY: Routledge.

Essen-Moeller, E. (1946). The concept of schizoidia. *Monatschrift für Psychiatrie und Neurologie, 112*, 258–271.

Esterberg, M. L. (2010). Cluster A personality disorders: Schizotypal, schizoid, and paranoid personality disorders in childhood and adolescence. *Journal of Psychopathology and Behavioral Assessment, 32*(4), 515–528.

Fairbairn, R. (1952). *Psychoanalytic studies of the personality*. London: Tavistock.

Guntrip, H. (1969). *Schizoid phenomena, object-relations, and the self*. New York, NY: International Universities Press.

Horney, K. (1999). *Neurosis and human growth: The struggle towards self-realization*. New York, NY: Routledge.

Jenkins, R. L., & Glickman, S. (1946). The schizoid child. *American Journal of Orthopsychiatry, 16*(2), 255–261.

Kraepelin, E. (1919). *Dementia praecox and paraphrenia* (R. M. Barclay, Trans.). Edinburgh: Livingstone.

Kretschmer, E. (1925). *Physique and character: An investigation of the nature of constitution and of the theory of temperament* (W. J. H. Sprott, Trans.). London: Kegan Paul, Trench & Trubner.

Kretschmer, E. (1931). *Physique and character*. London: Routledge (International Library of Psychology, 1999).

Laing, R. D. (1965). *The divided self: An existential study in sanity and madness*. Baltimore, MD: Penguin Books.

Livesley, W. J. (2003). *Practical management of personality disorder*. New York, NY: The Guilford Press.

Livesley, W. J., & West, M. (1986). The DSM-III distinction between schizoid and avoidant personality disorders. *Canadian Journal of Psychiatry, 31*(1), 59–62.

Martens, W. H. J. (2010). Schizoid personality disorder linked to unbearable and inescapable loneliness. *The European Journal of Psychiatry, 24*(1). doi:10.4321/S0213-61632010000100005

Masterson, J. F., & Klein, R. (1995). *Disorders of the self—The Masterson approach*. New York, NY: Brunner/Mazel.

Mather, A. A. (2008). Associations between body weight and personality disorders in a nationally representative sample. *Psychosomatic Medicine, 70*(9), 1012–1019.

MedlinePlus. (2014). Schizoid personality disorder. *National Library of Medicine*. Retrieved from https://www.nlm.nih.gov/medlineplus/ency/article/000920.htm

Millon, T. (2004). *Personality disorders in modern life* (2nd ed., pp. 371–374). New York, NY: Wiley.

Mittal, V. A., Kalus, O., Bernstein, D. P., & Siever, L. J. (2007). Schizoid personality disorder. In W. O'Donahue, K. A. Fowler, & S. O. Lilienfeld (Eds.), *Handbook of personality disorders: Toward the DSM-IV* (pp. 63–79). Thousand Oaks, CA: Sage Publications.

Mulder, R. T., Joyce, P. R., Frampton, C. M., Luty, S. E., & Sullivan, P. F. (2006). Six months of treatment for depression: Outcome and predictors of the course of illness. *The American Journal of Psychiatry, 163*, 95–100.

Nannarello, J. J. (1953). Schizoid. *The Journal of Nervous and Mental Disease, 118*(3), 237–249.

Panagiotis, P. (2012). A critique on the use of standard psychopathological classifications in understanding human distress: The example of "Schizoid Personality Disorder." *Counselling Psychology Review, 27*(1), 44–52.

Psychology Today. (2017). Schizoid personality disorder. Retrieved January 8, 2018, from https://www.psychologytoday.com/conditions/schizoid-personality-disorder

Rasmussen, P. R. (2005). The schizoid prototype. In *Personality-guided cognitive-behavioral therapy* (pp. 73–87). Washington, D.C.: American Psychological Association.

Rodriguez, Solano J. J., & De Chavez, M. G. (2000). Premorbid personality disorders in schizophrenia. *Schizophrenia Research, 44*(20), 137–144.

Rouff, L. (2000). Schizoid personality traits among the homeless mentally ill: A quantitative and qualitative report. *Journal of Social Distress and the Homeless, 9*(2), 127–141.

Seinfeld, J. (1991). *The empty core: An object relations approach to psychotherapy of the schizoid personality*. Lanham, MD: Jason Aronson.

Skodol, B. (2011). Personality disorder types proposal for DSM-5. *Journal of Personality Disorders, 25*(2), 150.

Triebwasser, J., Chemerinski, E., Roussos, P., & Siever, L. J. (2012). Schizoid personality disorder. *Journal of Personality Disorders, 26*(6), 919–926.

University of Colorado Springs (2001). An empirical investigation of Jung's personality types and psychological disorder-features. (http://www.cues.edu/Documents/dsegal/An0empirical-investigation-Jungs-types-and-PD-features-JPTT 2.pdf). *Journal of Psychological Type/University of Colorado Springs, 2001*. Retrieved August 10, 2013.

Winnicott, D. (2008). *The family and individual development*. New York, NY: Routledge.

Winnicott, D. (2012). *Playing and reality*. New York, NY: Routledge Classics.

Wolff, S. (1995). *Loners: The life path of unusual children*. London: Routledge.

Wood, J. (2017). Loneliness epidemic growing into biggest threat to public health. *Psych Central*. Retrieved September 13, 2017, from psychcentral.com

CHAPTER 10

Schizotypal Personality Disorder

Symptoms, Diagnosis, and Incidence

Schizotypal personality disorder's essential features have been described as a pervasive pattern of social and interpersonal deficits, accompanied by acute discomfort with, and reduced capacity for, close relationships as well as by cognitive or perceptual distortions and eccentricities of behavior. Beginning in early adulthood, this pattern is present in a variety of contexts (DSM-V, 2013).

Schizotypal personality disorder (STPD) is the most impairing disorder in Cluster A ("odd or eccentric disorders"; Comer & Comer, 2017). It occupies the middle of a spectrum of related disorders, with schizoid personality disorder being on the milder end and schizophrenia on the more severe end. It is thought that these disorders are probably biologically related and share similar genetic vulnerabilities.

Individuals suffering from this disorder often experience cognitive and perceptual distortions as well as eccentricities in their everyday behavior. Their difficulty in thinking and perceiving like other people intensifies their desire to avoid human interaction (Bayer, 2000).

Individuals with STPD often tend to incorrectly interpret casual incidents and external events as having an unusual meaning for them (ideas of reference). They may be superstitious or preoccupied with paranormal phenomena that are not part of their subculture. The feeling of special powers may lead them to believe that they can read others' thoughts or sense events before they actually happen, along with having the power to control others, either directly or indirectly, through complying with magical rituals. The speech of those with STPD is often digressive or vague, including unusual or idiosyncratic phrasing and construction.

Their verbal responses can be either overly concrete or overly abstract, with words or concepts sometimes being applied in unusual ways.

People with this disorder are often suspicious, believing some people (colleagues or personal acquaintances) are trying to undermine their reputation with others. Individuals with STPD are frequently considered odd or eccentric due to their unusual mannerisms, an unkempt manner of dress, and inattention to the usual conventions.

In general, interpersonal relatedness seems problematic for people with STPD due to their discomfort in relating to other people. As a result, they have no or just a few close friends or confidants other than first-degree relatives. They are usually anxious in social situations, especially those involving unfamiliar people; and because their anxiety seems to be associated with suspiciousness regarding other people's motives, the anxiety remains even as time goes on and their acquaintances become more familiar. The schizotypal person does not become more relaxed with passing time.

At times schizotypal individuals interpret situations as being strange or having unusual meaning for them. They often seek medical attention for anxiety or depression instead of their personality disorder (DSM-5, 2013).

Reported prevalence rates in community studies of STPD range from 0.6 percent in Norwegian samples to 4.6 percent in a U.S. community sample. In clinical populations the prevalence of STPD seems to be infrequent (0%–1.9%), with a higher estimated prevalence in the general population (3.9%), according to the National Epidemiologic Survey on Alcohol and Related Conditions, whereas the DSM-IV reported a lower—almost 3 percent—occurrence within the general population. STPD may be slightly more common in males than in females. It can first appear in childhood or adolescence as strange fantasies, social anxiety, hypersensitivity, or other odd behavior. Together with other Cluster A personality disorders, STPD is also quite common among homeless people (Connolly, 2008).

STPD often co-occurs with major depressive disorder, dysthymia, and generalized social phobia (Adams & Sutker, 2001). It also can sometimes co-occur with obsessive-compulsive disorder, where it can adversely affect treatment outcome. The list of personality disorders that co-occur most often with STPD includes schizoid, paranoid, avoidant, and borderline personality disorders (Tasman et al., 2008).

STPD's high rate of comorbidity with other personality disorders may be due to overlapping criteria with other personality disorders, such as avoidant personality disorder, paranoid personality disorder, and borderline personality disorder (McGlashan et al., 2000).

The World Health Organization's *ICD-10*—using the name *schizo-typal disorder*—has classified STPD as a clinical disorder associated with schizophrenia, rather than a personality disorder as in *DSM-5*.

Timeline

1956   Sandor Rado coined the term *schizotype* as an abbreviation of *schizophrenic phenotype*.
2004   Theodore Millon identified two subtypes of schizotypal personality disorder.

History

American psychiatrist Sandor Rado first suggested the term *schizotype* for the behavioral and psychodynamic expression of a genetic predisposition to schizophrenia. He thought that people genetically predisposed to schizophrenia might be stable in their adaptation to life. He labeled them *schizoid* in the sense that Kraepelin and Bleuler used the term. Rado applied the term *schizotypal* if such predisposed people displayed more florid symptoms.

Since then, the term *schizotypy* has been used for the personality disorder that shows the clearest genetic relationship to schizophrenia, although it is often associated with schizoid and paranoid personality disorders. It is the personality disorder most often found in close relatives of schizophrenic patients.

Attempting to provide a historical perspective on the *DSM-III* concept of STPD, it was pointed out that the conceptualization of this diagnostic entity was influenced by two major traditions (Kendler, 1985). One of these approaches, the *familial* approach, underlines the characteristic traits found in the deviant but nonpsychotic relatives of schizophrenics. The focus of the second, the *clinical* approach, was on patients who seem to demonstrate the fundamental symptoms of schizophrenia—however, without psychotic symptoms or severe personality deterioration. Reviewing these two traditions, it was determined that they are similar in some regards, but there are also important differences in their views regarding the characteristics of the true "schizotype." Both of these traditions can be expected to influence relevant research efforts in this general area, as for example, the Danish Adoption Studies linked to the development of the *DSM-III* criteria for schizotypal personality.

Theodore Millon (2004) proposed two subtypes of STPD: insipid schizotypal, which is thought to be a structural exaggeration of the passive-detached pattern, including schizoid, depressive, and dependent features; and timorous schizotypal, which is viewed as a structural exaggeration of the active-detached pattern, including avoidant and negativistic features. Any individual with STPD may exhibit either one of the somewhat different subtypes.

The *ICD-10* calls this disorder schizotypal disorder and equates it with "latent" or "borderline" schizophrenia rather than with personality disorders.

Development and Causes

Although there are many theories about the possible causes of STPD, many professionals seem to prescribe to a biopsychosocial model of causation (Bressert, 2017). Others consider STPD to be a "schizophrenia spectrum" disorder. Schizophrenia is considered to have a genetic basis, which, in turn, suggests that STPD shares the same genetic etiology (Nigg & Goldsmith, 1994).

Occurrence rates of this disorder are much higher in relatives of individuals with schizophrenia than in the relatives of people with other mental illnesses or in those without mentally ill relatives. Being considered an "extended phenotype" schizotypal personality disorder can be an aid to geneticists tracking the familial or genetic transmission of the genes that are implicated in schizophrenia (Fogelson et al., 2007). In addition, there seems to be a genetic connection of STPD to mood disorders, particularly depression (Comer & Comer, 2017).

Having a family history of mental illness constitutes a risk factor for developing STPD. People who have first-degree relatives with schizotypal symptoms (schizotypy) can be as much as 50 percent more likely to develop schizotypy compared to people without that family history. Those who have a close relative with schizophrenia may also be more likely to develop STPD and to experience symptoms of similar severity to their schizophrenic relative. Also, medical conditions such as epilepsy can be a predisposing factor to developing schizotypy as an adult (WebMed, 2017).

STPD is the personality disorder found in the closest relatives of schizophrenic patients, more often in identical twins than in nonidentical twins of schizophrenic patients. Also, it occurs more often in biological rather than in the adoptive parents of schizophrenics (McGuffin & Thapar, 1992).

Evidence shows that the Cluster A group of schizotypal, schizoid, and paranoid personality disorders are all biologically related to schizophrenia (Varma & Sharma, 1993). Evidence also suggests that parenting styles, early separation, and trauma/maltreatment history can lead to the development of schizotypal traits (Anglina, Cohenab, & Chena, 2008). The risk of developing STPD is increased by such occurrences as neglect or abuse, trauma, or family dysfunction during childhood. In general, children learn to interpret social cues over time and respond appropriately, but for unknown reasons, for people with this disorder, this process does not work well (Mayo Clinic Staff, 2012).

It has been observed that children raised by schizophrenic parents have a greater probability of developing STPD than children raised by parents without a mental impairment. The process of developing the disorder has been described with the child observing and emulating the schizophrenic parent's behavior. And it is equally likely that the schizophrenic parent would encourage the development of the child's "magical" paranormal belief because the parent is convinced that the child possesses these paranormal skills. This developmental process of magical thinking is further illustrated when contemplating situations where evangelistic children allegedly can heal by laying on of hands. Possibly being raised by a schizophrenic parent, the child is told that he or she possesses special powers. Reinforcing the child's beliefs in the possession of these paranormal skills at the same time reinforces the schizophrenic parent's delusions regarding the child's possession of these skills. The combination of modeled behavior and reinforced beliefs predispose the child's development of STPD (Dobbert, 2007).

Among possible social risk factors for developing the suspiciousness and unusual perceptive symptoms of STPD are birth during the winter or summer, higher birth order, being the victim of childhood physical or sexual abuse, or having a lower family socioeconomic status during childhood. Apparently, it has also been found to occur more often in black women compared to other women, independent of socioeconomic factors. Parents who have difficulty communicating or who tend to engage in magical thinking, such as purporting what their children are thinking, also may present risk factors for children growing up to develop STPD. Still other risk factors apparently have been noted with children who use marijuana for the first time before 14 years of age or who have been prematurely placed in the role of an adult (WebMed, 2017).

If people with STPD are intellectually gifted, they may strive toward achievements, and this may be helpful in compensating for their emotional deficiencies (Rado, 1954).

Effects and Costs

The social consequences of a serious mental disorder like STPD, a disorder that affects a person's ability to function in social and occupational settings, can be calamitous. A common attention impairment in various degrees characterizing STPD could serve as a marker of biological susceptibility to STPD. The reason for this occurrence is that an individual having difficulty with taking in information may face problems in complicated social situations where interpersonal cues and attentive communications are essential for quality interaction. Eventually, this might cause the individual to withdraw from most social interactions, leading to asociality (Lees Roitman et al., 1997).

Schizotypal individuals' perceptual alterations may include hearing someone whispering his or her name even though no other person is present. Rising paranoid ideation might make the schizotypal person fear that fellow employees are secretly talking and laughing about him or her, which would likely lead to difficulties at work and eventually loss of his or her job. Additionally, schizotypal persons usually do not respond properly to interpersonal cues (Bayer, 2000). They may avoid eye contact, appear unkempt, exhibit unusual mannerisms, or dress inappropriately. These characteristics are not only provoking negative judgment in social situations but in work settings as well.

The tension, anxiety, and suspicion people with STPD experience in so many of their interactions with others may eventually lead to depression. If severely depressed for a long period of time, transient psychotic episodes can occur. In clinical settings, between 30 percent and 50 percent of schizotypal patients have also been diagnosed as suffering from a major depressive disorder (Bayer, 2000). Many individuals having this personality disorder in addition to another mental disorder were observed to be less responsive to treatment.

It has been found that individuals with STPD who use methamphetamine are at great risk of developing permanent psychosis (Chen et al., 2005).

STPD can easily be confused with schizophrenia, a severe mental illness. But while people with STPD may experience brief psychotic episodes with hallucinations or delusions, these episodes are less frequent, prolonged, or intense than in schizophrenia. Another important distinction can be seen in the fact that individuals with STPD usually can be made aware of the difference between their distorted ideas and reality. Those suffering from schizophrenia generally cannot be swayed away from their delusions (Mayo Clinic, 2017a).

Factors most likely beneficial in reducing the symptoms of this disorder are positive relationships with friends and family and a sense of achievement at school, work, and in extracurricular activities (Mayo Clinic, 2017b).

In Society

People with STPD, much like schizoid patients, do not respond properly to interpersonal cues. They appear stiff or rigid emotionally and exhibit eccentric behavior that does not fit in with the rest of society. They may look unkempt or dress inappropriately, ignore social conventions, avoid eye contact, or display unusual mannerisms (Wood, 2010). Individuals with this disorder also tend to have markedly illogical thinking, with odd beliefs or unusual ideas that are not consistent with prevailing ideas held by the general public. In addition, they may report unusual perceptions or strange body experiences that other people might have difficulty comprehending.

STPD shares many similarities with schizoid personality disorder; most notably among them is the inability to initiate or maintain relationships (both friendly and romantic). However, there is a difference between the two disorders when it comes to the reason for the relationship difficulties: schizotypal individuals avoid social interaction because of a deep-seated fear or distrust of people, while schizoid individuals are not interested in forming relationships because they have no desire to share their time with others.

Considering some of the diagnostic criteria for STPD, such as odd thinking and speech, ideas of reference, odd beliefs or magical thinking, suspiciousness or paranoid thinking, inappropriate or constricted affect, odd or eccentric appearance or behavior, and excessive social anxiety, among others, it is not difficult to understand that these individuals experience significant problems in interactions with others and that they would rather avoid any such experiences.

"Unabomber" Ted Kaczynski is believed to be an extreme example of STPD. For almost two decades, his eccentric beliefs of protecting the world led him to send homemade pipe bombs to academic and business leaders in the computer and technology fields (Diamond, 2008).

Up Close
Carole's mother is worried because 19-year-old Carole is withdrawn and seems to have no real friends. Carole does not talk much, and when she

does, her poor social skills become apparent. Also, her mind seems to be operating on the periphery of any social interaction, as if she does not quite understand the exact content of conversations. She did not do well in school, partly due to her high anxiety and partly because of her unusual behaviors. Currently Carole is enrolled in a vocational school, trying to find out what work activities she could perform in the future. But here, again, she has great difficulty "fitting in."

Most of Carole's free time is spent on the computer, playing online games, making up somewhat bizarre stories about herself when interacting with others in chat rooms, and visiting Web sites that advertise paranormal research and experiences. Carole steadfastly believes in ghosts, and from time to time, she reports hearing strange noises.

Carole's behavior reminds her mother of her own sister, who has been diagnosed with schizophrenia. Will Carole end up like her aunt? her mother worries.

At Work

The eccentric behaviors and odd speech exhibited by people with STPD can be expected to lead to distraction and misunderstandings in most work situations. Combined with these individuals' suspiciousness and inappropriate display of feelings, it is not difficult to foresee difficulties in the work place. And, in turn, schizotypal people's tendency toward "magical thinking" not only impacts their perceptions of reality but also may lead to cognitive distortion and misinterpretations of their environment as well as their coworkers' behaviors.

Routine interactions at work may be very awkward and anxiety provoking for schizotypal individuals. However, they may be more capable of performing jobs that are well structured and require little, if any, social interaction. It would also be helpful if a job supervisor could understand and accommodate the person's eccentricities (Harvard Medical School, 2013).

Their excessive social anxiety does not diminish with familiarity and tends to be associated with paranoid fears rather than with negative judgments about oneself. That means that over time, the anxiety of those with STPD about their coworkers remains as high as if they just met for the first time. And if there is any negativity associated with interactions, individuals with STPD do not look at themselves or their behavior as a possible reason for any negative aspects; their suspicion toward the other person increases immediately (Bressert, 2017).

Up Close

It took Nathan several years to find a job he was able to hold for longer than a month. He grew up as an only child and spent much time by himself after school as both his parents worked. He developed a peculiar way of talking, and the other children at school teased him, which made him angry, but usually he was too afraid to express it openly because he interpreted their teasing as more severely threatening than it actually was. Nathan hated school and tried to play sick as often as he could get away with. Although of average intelligence, Nathan's grades were pitiful, mainly because of his many absences. He barely graduated from high school.

During the time he spent alone at home, Nathan learned to fix himself snacks and sandwiches, developing an interest in cooking. Fortunately, the local community college offered a program leading to a certificate in culinary arts. Nathan managed to be accepted provisionally because of his poor high school standing. His social skills had not improved, and he remained a loner through the time of his community college attendance. An added difficulty arose from Nathan's tendency to at times insist on making up his own recipes instead of following the teacher's instructions.

An important part of the culinary program consisted of a practical experience, an apprenticeship at local restaurants. Each student was assigned to a hotel or restaurant for this practicum. Nathan's occupational path did not survive the apprenticeship. After several weeks of spending this part of his education at a mid-class restaurant, the owner complained to the community college, terminating Nathan's apprenticeship. According to the complaint, Nathan seemed to have difficulty understanding parts of the culinary processes—at times, when not closely observed, changing the course of cooking events, turning the planned menu items into haphazard culinary expressions. In addition, he had problems communicating with the rest of the staff in comprehensible ways. As Nathan's admission to the community college had been on a provisional basis, the apprenticeship failure led straight to Nathan's dismissal from the community college.

Nathan's next ill-fated attempt at finding a workplace was to apply as a server in a local fast-food restaurant. Although it was not difficult to expect another failure, considering Nathan's poor social skills, he still did not want to let go of his culinary interests and apparently hoped for another chance in this area. In fact, he tried several short-lived jobs at different restaurants before finally giving up.

He applied at local warehouses, where his physical strength was an asset. But sooner or later, he ran into difficulties with coworkers because of his eccentric way of communication or occasional outbursts of anger. Wherever he worked, he remained a loner, never associating with coworkers during breaks because he did not trust anyone.

His parents were concerned. Nathan's mother saw some of his father's poor communication skills and tendency to withdraw from others in Nathan's personality. As she recognized those traits in the two men in her family, she remembered seeing a commercial on TV, advertising the services of a truck driver training organization. She prepared herself with paper and pencil for the next time the commercial came on the air and wrote down the information. She shared the information with her husband but not with Nathan. She needed to check out the business before telling Nathan about it and applying for the training. As a result of this process Nathan became a long-distance truck driver with a steady route and minimal required verbal communication.

In Relationships

Individuals with STPD typically have few, if any, close friends, and they feel nervous around strangers, but they may marry and maintain jobs. However, the extreme discomfort experienced by schizotypal individuals within close relationships will most often not permit the development of intimacy and openness. For some, their difficulty with creating close relationships is related to their eccentric habits. And as emotional closeness does not increase with familiarity and passage of time, there is little hope that a marital relationship with a schizotypal partner would develop the level of closeness other spouses in normal marriages strive for.

Experts' repeated mention of schizotypal individuals' lack of close friends or confidants other than first-degree relatives would seem to make it impossible for them to enter into or remain for long in an intimate romantic relationship, as passage of time apparently does not increase the level of personal openness of the schizotypal individual.

Up Close

This was moving day for 34-year-old Donald. His wife, Janet, moved out a week ago and filed for divorce, The condominium was nice but too big for him, and Janet did not want to stay in town. In her disappointment about their marriage, she decided on a big geographical move. Donald was moving back to his mother's home; it seemed like a reasonable solution.

Janet's complaint was mostly about Donald's emotional coldness. After the initial attraction, she did not know how to relate to him. He did not express warm feelings and did not tell her much about himself. It was difficult to know what he liked. His work in information technology seemed to explain Donald's fascination with computers. He not only spent his work hours with them but most of his time at home, too.

When he had to travel on business, Donald never called Janet at home to find out how she felt and how she spent her time. Janet felt lonely and neglected; she missed the intimacy she had expected to find in her marriage. And she could not imagine raising children with Donald.

Theory and Research

STPD is thought to be influenced by biology, psychology, and social and cultural factors. Social anxiety and isolation are core elements of this disorder. Researchers suggest that this personality disorder may share some genetic basis with schizophrenia.

Biological influences indicate a genetic vulnerability for schizophrenia but without the biological or environmental stresses present in that disorder. Social/cultural influences can be seen in the preference for social isolation, excessive social anxiety, and lack of social skills. Psychological influences include unusual beliefs, behavior, or dress; the belief that insignificant events are personally relevant ("ideas of reference"); reduced or lack of emotional expression; and symptoms of major depressive disorder. All these influences are thought to combine for the development of STPD.

In order to provide an instrument for the assessment of STPD that would address all nine schizotypal traits, the Schizotypal Personality Disorder Questionnaire (SPQ) was developed as a self-report scale, modeled on the relevant *DSM-III-R* criteria. The questionnaire, consisting of nine subscales, was evaluated for effectiveness in a study involving two samples of normal subjects (n = 302 and n = 195) to test the replicability of findings (Raine, 1991).

The SPQ was found to have high sampling validity, high internal reliability (0.91), test-retest reliability (0.82), convergent validity (0.59 to 0.81), discriminant validity and criterion validity (0.63, 0.68). The findings were replicated across samples. Fifty-five percent of subjects scoring in the top 10 percent of SPQ scores had a clinical diagnosis of STPD. The results would indicate the SPQ's usefulness in screening for STPD in the general population as well as in researching the correlates of individual schizotypal traits.

Some information-processing measures serve as biological markers for schizophrenia, and they can also help in defining the boundaries of schizophrenia. Prepulse inhibition and habituation of the blink reflex component of startle, which are believed to reflect an individual's ability to screen out or "gate" irrelevant sensory stimuli, are impaired in patients with schizophrenia. It was hypothesized that individuals with STPD would show a loss of sensorimotor gating, reflected by impaired prepulse inhibition of the human startle response, and that they would show deficits in startle habituation consistent with the deficits observed in patients with schizophrenia (Cadenhead, Geyer, & Braff, 1993).

To test the hypotheses, prepulse inhibition and habituation were assessed in 12 men and 4 women who met *DSM-III-R* criteria for STPD and in 22 normal comparison subjects. The results revealed that patients with STPD had deficits in acoustic prepulse inhibition and habituation similar to the deficits seen in patients with schizophrenia. There were no differences noted between patients with STPD and normal subjects in the latency from acoustic startle stimuli to a response, but latency facilitation was produced by the prepulse in both groups.

The investigators concluded that this pattern of changes in amplitude and latency of the startle response suggests that individuals with STPD perceive the prepulse stimuli but still show deficient sensorimotor gating of amplitude. These findings demonstrate the importance of startle prepulse inhibition and startle habituation as biological markers for schizophreniform spectrum disorders.

In a later study, researchers hypothesized that nonschizophrenic relatives of patients with schizophrenia would also have prepulse inhibition deficits, which would indicate a genetically transmitted susceptibility to sensorimotor gating deficits (Cadenhead, Swerdlow, Shafer, Diaz, & Braff, 2000b). In this study 23 patients with schizophrenia, 34 relatives of schizophrenic patients, 11 individuals with STPD, and 25 comparison subjects were assessed in an acoustic startle paradigm. The eye-blink component of the startle response was evaluated bilaterally through electromyographic recordings of orbicularis oculi. Reduced prepulse inhibition was observed in patients with schizophrenia, their relatives, and subjects with STPD relative to the comparison subjects. These deficits were more evident in measures of right eye-blink prepulse inhibition. The comparison subjects demonstrated greater right versus left eye-blink prepulse inhibition, while the probands, their relatives, and subjects with STPD showed less asymmetry of prepulse inhibition.

It was concluded that the data suggested a genetically transmitted deficit in prepulse inhibition (sensorimotor gating) in patients with schizophrenia spectrum disorders, including individuals with STPD and relatives of patients with schizophrenia. In addition, the reduced prepulse inhibition in subjects with STPD indicated that prepulse inhibition is a potentially useful neurobiological marker for intermediate phenotypes of schizophrenia spectrum disorders.

Individuals in the schizophrenia spectrum have difficulties with attention, cognition, and information processing. It is possible to assess the functions of attention and information processing by testing suppression of the P50 event-related potential. The amplitude of the P50 wave is measured in response to each of two auditory clicks. In normal individuals, the P50 wave following the second click is suppressed or "gated." But in schizophrenic patients and their relatives, there is less suppression of the second P50 wave. There is a high heritability for deficits in P50 suppression, and it shows a linkage to the alpha-7 subunit of the nicotinic cholinergic receptor gene in families with schizophrenia, suggesting that deficits in P50 suppression are trait markers for gating abnormalities in schizophrenia spectrum subjects.

It has been noted that schizotypal individuals have deficits in sensorimotor gating as measured by prepulse inhibition, but P50 sensory gating in individuals with schizotypal personality disorder has not been reported yet (Cadenhead, Light, Geyer, & Braff, 2000a). In a study involving 26 individuals with STPD and 23 normal subjects, P50 suppression was assessed through auditory conditioning and testing. The results showed that the individuals with STPD had significantly less P50 suppression than the normal subjects. It was concluded that individuals with STPD may have trait-linked sensory gating deficits, similar to those in patients with schizophrenia and their relatives. Because sensory gating deficits were observed in those subjects without overt psychotic symptoms, it seems likely that these deficits represent a core cognitive dysfunction of the schizophrenia spectrum (Cadenhead et al., 2000a).

Clues to the question of diagnostic boundaries of schizophrenic spectrum categories were found in the aggregation of disorders in families identified by a schizophrenic disorder proband (index case). The Danish Adoption Studies provided quasi-experimental evidence for the range of expression of a putative schizophrenic spectrum disorder, which was later denoted STPD in *DSM-III-R* (Squires-Wheeler, Skodol, Bassett, & Erlenmeyer-Kimling, 1989). The hypothesis had been that such schizophrenic spectrum categories have a genetic relationship to schizophrenic disorder and, therefore, form a continuum with schizophrenia in terms of etiology and pathogenesis. In order to be able to make meaningful use of such spectrum categories in genetic analyses (e.g., linkage analysis), it is necessary for rates of spectrum traits and disorder in normal control and in psychiatric control populations to be known.

Three offspring groups (ages 18–29) defined by parental diagnoses, including schizophrenic disorder (n = 90), affective disorder (n = 79), and no parental disorder (n = 161), were used to assess the rate of *DSM-III-R* schizotypal traits and disorder. Trained social workers and psychologists conducted the assessment. The rates of three, four, and five schizotypal features were evaluated in the offspring with parental psychiatric disorder in contrast to the offspring with no parental psychiatric disorder. Because the rates between the offspring of the schizophrenic disorder parental group and the offspring of the affective disorder parental group did not differ significantly, support for the assumption of diagnostic specificity for those categories was not confirmed.

Questions about the relationship between schizophrenia and STPD as defined in *DSM-III* prompted another independent analysis of the Copenhagen Sample of the Danish Adoption Study of Schizophrenia (Kendler, Gruenberg, & Strauss, 1981). As the interviews of relatives from the study were independently and blindly reevaluated (as described in the above article), it was found that the prevalence of STPD was significantly higher in the biological relatives of the schizophrenic adoptees than in the biological relatives of matched controls and was low and equal in the two groups of adoptive relatives. Compared with "borderline" and uncertain borderline schizophrenia, the criteria for STPD were more specific but less sensitive in identifying biologic relatives of schizophrenics. As demonstrated in this sample, STPD appears to have a strong genetic, but no familial-environmental relationship to schizophrenia. These results constitute a validation of the diagnosis of STPD.

Although STPD aggregates in relatives of schizophrenic probands, researchers have raised the issue that the criteria for this disorder may not be optimal either in describing the dimensions of schizotypal phenomena or in identifying those with a high familial liability to schizophrenia (Kendler et al., 1995). As part of the Roscommon Family Study, an epidemiologically based family study of major psychiatric disorders conducted in the west of Ireland, researchers examined 25 individual schizotypal symptoms and signs through the use of structured personal interviews with 1,544 first-degree relatives (without chronic psychosis or mental retardation) of five proband groups: schizophrenia; other nonaffective psychoses; psychotic affective illness; nonpsychotic affective illness; and matched, unscreened controls.

The following seven meaningful schizotypal factors were obtained: negative schizotypy, positive schizotypy, borderline symptoms, social dysfunction, avoidant symptoms, odd speech, and suspicious behavior. Except for borderline symptoms, all these factors significantly discriminated relatives of schizophrenic probands from relatives of controls. Schizotypal factors differed in their specificity. In addition, three of the four most predictive schizotypal factors significantly discriminated relatives of probands with other nonaffective psychoses from relatives of controls.

The researchers considered "schizotypy" to be a complex, multidimensional construct, whose various dimensions differ widely both in degree and specificity with which they reflect the familial liability to schizophrenia.

Investigations into the type and nature of personality disorders among biological relatives of schizophrenic probands involved a total of 176 nonschizophrenic co-twins and other first-degree relatives of schizophrenic probands in comparison to 101 co-twins and first-degree relatives of probands with major depression. It was found that schizotypal personality disorders were more common and histrionic personality disorders less common among the biological relatives of schizophrenic probands than among relatives of probands with major depression. Furthermore, the so-called "negative" schizotypal criteria like odd speech, inappropriate affect, and odd behavior, as well as excessive social anxiety, were significantly more common among the relatives of schizophrenic probands. The so-called "positive" schizotypal criteria were partly, but not statistically significantly, more common among the relatives of probands with major depression. The differences in frequencies of the negative criteria between monozygotic co-twins, dizygotic co-twins, and other first-degree relatives of schizophrenic probands were insignificant. It was concluded that *DSM-III-R* schizotypal disorder is defined by a set of criteria that partly describe a "true" schizophrenia-related personality disorder and partly features that are not specific for relatives of schizophrenic probands. In addition, the genetic relationship between schizophrenia and "true" STPD appears weak. A marker of a possible genetic link between the disorders may be excessive social anxiety (Torgersen, Onstad, Skre, Edvardsen, & Kringlen, 1993).

Earlier evidence suggests that personality disorders include a significant genetic component as most of the early studies explored the disorder's frequency in the relatives of individuals diagnosed with Cluster A disorders (as well as borderline and antisocial personality disorders). However, the assumption of a genetic basis is not conclusive because family studies cannot disentangle genetic and environmental factors because either one of them—or a combination of both—could account for the disorder's increased incidence in the relatives of affected individuals. Furthermore, psychosocial theories of causation also predict an increased occurrence in family members. Twin or adoption studies are needed to separate genetic and environmental contributing factors. Twin studies are the vehicle to provide convincing evidence for a genetic basis to personality disorders. However, in general, the focus of these twin studies has been on personality traits rather than on personality disorders (Livesley, 2001).

In an evaluation of 29 obsessive-compulsive patients for behavior therapy, 10 of them (35%) had Axis II diagnosis of STPD. Of the patients without the diagnosis of STPD, 16 (84%) improved at least moderately with either behavior therapy alone or a combination of behavior therapy and pharmacotherapy. Among the STPD group, only one (10%) improved with the same treatment. This difference was highly significant, emphasizing the level of impairments within the patient groups (Minichiello, 1987).

Some individuals with STPD may develop schizophrenia, but the majority do not (Raine, 2006). As STPD symptomatology has been studied longitudinally in several community samples, the results do not suggest any significant likelihood of the development of schizophrenia (Gooding, Tallent, & Matts, 2005).

Many studies show that individuals with STPD score similar to individuals with schizophrenia on a very wide range of neuropsychological tests. Also, cognitive deficits in patients with STPD are quite similar to, but not the same as, those in patients with schizophrenia, thus agreeing with the observations of a 2004 study, which reported neurological evidence that did not completely support the notion that STPD is simply an attenuated form of schizophrenia (Haznedar et al., 2004).

In a cohort of patients with major depressive disorder undergoing a 6-month treatment, it was found that the presence of symptoms of STPD was linked to poorer treatment outcome (Mulder, Joyce, Frampton, Luty, & Sullivan, 2006).

In a study comparing psychosocial functioning in patients with schizotypal, borderline, avoidant, or obsessive-compulsive personality disorder; patients with major depressive disorder; and no personality disorder, it was hypothesized that the degree of associated functional impairment would differ among the personality disorders and that patients with severe (i.e., schizotypal or borderline) personality disorders would show more functional impairment than patients with less severe (i.e., avoidant or obsessive-compulsive) personality disorders or with major depressive disorder (Skodol et al., 2002).

A comparison of the mean levels of impairment in psychosocial functioning during the month before intake for the different patient groups revealed that patients with STPD and borderline personality disorder consistently exhibited greater functional impairment than patients with obsessive-compulsive disorder or major depressive disorder.

On self-report measures regarding impairment for the two weeks before assessment, the results were consistent with the interview ratings. Patients with STPD and borderline personality disorder rated themselves as significantly more impaired on all individual domains of functioning and overall than those with obsessive-compulsive personality disorder and major depressive disorder. Patients with avoidant personality disorder were in the intermediate range.

Individuals with Cluster A personality disorder (paranoid, schizoid, and schizotypal) have a 10 times greater chance of having three or more Axis I disorders than individuals without a personality disorder (Bjornlund, 2011).

A study investigating the effect of comorbid personality disorders on the perceived stress in depressed patients suggested that individuals with STPD prototypically exhibit a pervasive pattern of social and interpersonal deficits characterized by discomfort with close relationships, which might function as a specific link between Cluster A comorbidity and stress appraisal (Candrian et al., 2008).

Comparing personality disorders and Myers-Briggs Type Indicator types in a University of Colorado, Colorado Springs study found that STPD had a significant correlation with the Introverted (I), Intuitive (N), Thinking (T), and Perceiving (P) preferences.

Treatment

In cases where a person's symptoms are mild to moderate, he or she may be able to adjust with relatively little support. Those with more severe problems, however, may have more than average difficulty maintaining a job or living independently, and they may need more support from family members. Those who are severely afflicted with the disorder may need hospitalization to provide therapy and improve socialization. They do not often show significant progress, and some think that treatment goals should focus on helping patients establish a satisfying solitary existence.

There are no medications approved by the Food and Drug Administration specifically for the treatment of STPD, but antipsychotics, mood stabilizers, antidepressants, or antianxiety drugs may be prescribed to help relieve certain symptoms that are easily observable (Mayo Clinic, 2017b). For instance, illogical thinking can be treated with antipsychotic medications, usually in low doses, whereas depression or anxiety might respond to antidepressant or antianxiety medications (Harvard Medical School, 2013).

Although STPD may be one of the easiest personality disorders to identify, it is also one of the most difficult to treat with psychotherapy, according to Theodore Millon (2004). STPD patients may be able to benefit from behavioral modification, a cognitive-behavioral treatment approach, allowing them to understand how their thoughts and behaviors affect each other and remedy some of the bizarre thoughts and behaviors. Of particular importance is the improvement of social skills in addressing the long-standing social deficits that accompany STPD. Two effective methods of treatment are recognizing abnormalities by watching videotapes and meeting with a therapist to improve speech habits.

Unless groups are well structured and supportive, group therapy is not recommended for people suffering from STPD because the statements and references made by various group members it could lead to loose, tangential ideation within the individual with STPD (Livesley, 2001).

For schizotypal patients with predominant paranoid ideation, support is especially important because they usually have great difficulties even in highly structured groups. As mentioned above, in a clinical setting, these individuals are rarely seen for STPD-related reasons; mostly it occurs as a comorbid finding with other mental disorders. In cases where patients with STPD are prescribed medication, they are often the same drugs used to treat patients with schizophrenia, including traditional neuroleptics (Livesley, 2001). As mentioned earlier, antipsychotic medications in low doses can be helpful; through the careful choice of medications, many schizotypal patients are able to function adequately in the everyday world. And mainly because of drug therapy, the hospitalization length for such disorders has been greatly reduced (Bayer, 2000).

For people suffering from STPD, comprehensive treatment is crucial for symptom alleviation and for finding a path toward recovery. Formal treatment systems may be enhanced by consumer help programs, family self-help, advocacy, and services for housing as well as vocational assistance—all supplementing the formal treatment system. Treatment for this disorder is most effective when family members are involved and supportive. Many of these services are operated by mental health service recipients. The logic behind this arrangement is that those using the system might be especially effective in reaching out to those in need (Psychology Today, 2017).

References

Adams, H. E., & Sutker, P. B. (2001). *Comprehensive handbook of psychopathology* (3rd ed.). New York, NY: Springer.

Anglina, D. M., Cohenab, P. R., & Chena, H. (2008). Duration of early maternal separation and prediction of schizotypal symptoms from early adolescence to midlife. *Schizophrenia Research, 103*(1), 143–150.

Bayer, L. (2000). *Personality disorders.* Philadelphia, PA: Chelsea House Publishers.

Bjornlund, L. (2011). *Personality disorders.* San Diego, CA: Reference Point Press.

Bressert, S. (2017). Schizotypal personality disorder. *Psych Central.* Retrieved December 26, 2017, from https://psychocentral.com/disorders /schizotypal-personality-disorder/

Cadenhead, K. S., Geyer, M. A., & Braff, D. L. (1993). Impaired startle prepulse inhibition and habituation in patients with schizotypal personality disorder. *American Journal of Psychiatry, 150,* 1862–1867.

Cadenhead, K. S., Light, G., Geyer, M., & Braff, D. (2000a). Sensory gating deficits assessed by the P50 event-related-potential in subjects with schizotypal personality disorder. *American Journal of Psychiatry, 157,* 55–59.

Cadenhead, K. S., Swerdlow, N. R., Shafer, K. M., Diaz, M., & Braff, D. L. (2000b). Modulation of the startle response and startle laterality in relatives of schizophrenic patients and in subjects with schizotypal personality disorder: Evidence of inhibitory deficits. *American Journal of Psychiatry.* doi:10.1176/appi.ajp.157.10.1660

Candrian, M., Schwartz, F., Farabaugh, A., Perlis, R. H., Ehlert, U., & Fava, M. (2008). Personality disorders and perceived stress in Major Depressive Disorder. *Psychiatry Research, 160*(2), 184–191.

Chen, C. K., Lin, S. K., Sham, P. C., Ball, D., Loh, E. W., Li, T., & Murray, R. M. (2005). Morbid risk for psychiatric disorder among the relatives of methamphetamine users with and without psychosis. *American Journal of Medical Genetics, 136*(1), 87–91.

Comer, R., & Comer, G. (2017). *Personality disorders.* Princeton, NJ: Worth Publishers.

Connolly, A. J. (2008). Personality disorders in homeless drop-in center clients. *Journal of Personality Disorders, 22*(6), 573–588.

Diamond, S. (2008). Terrorism, resentment, and the Unabomber. *Psychology Today*. Posted April 8, 2008. Psychologytoday.com

Dobbert, D. L. (2007). *Understanding personality disorders: An introduction*. Westport, CT: Praeger Publishers.

Fogelson, D. L., Nuechterlein, K. H., Asarnow, R. F., Payne, D. L., Subotnik, K. L., Jacobson, K. C., … Kendler, K. S. (2007). Avoidant personality disorder is a separable schizophrenia-spectrum personality disorder even when controlling for the presence of paranoid and schizotypal personality disorders: The UCLA family study. *Schizophrenia Research, 91*, 192–199.

Gooding, D. C., Tallent, K. A., & Matts, C. W. (2005). Clinical status of at-risk individuals 5 years later: Further validation of the psychometric high-risk strategy. *Journal of Abnormal Psychology, 114*(1), 170–175.

Harvard Medical School. (2013). Schizotypal personality disorder. *Harvard Health Publishing*. Retrieved June 1, 2018, from https://www.health.harvard.edu/mind-and-mood/schizotypal-personality-disorder-

Haznedar, M. M., Buchsbaum, M. S., Hazlett, E. A., Shihabuddin, L., New, A., & Siever, L. J. (2004). Cingulate gyrus volume and metabolism in the schizophrenia spectrum. *Schizophrenia Research, 71*(2–3), 249–262.

Healthline. (2018). Schizotypal personality disorder (STPD). Retrieved June 18, 2018, from https://www.healthline.com/health/schizotypal-personality-disorder

Kendler, K. S. (1985). Diagnostic approaches to schizotypal personality disorder: A historical perspective. *Schizophrenia Bulletin, 11*(4), 538–553.

Kendler, K. S., Gruenberg, A. M., & Strauss, J. S. (1981). An independent analysis of the Copenhagen Sample of the Danish Adoption Study of schizophrenia. II. The relationship between schizotypal personality disorder and schizophrenia. *Archives of General Psychiatry, 38*(9), 982–984.

Kendler, K. S., McGuire, M., Gruenberg, A. M., & Walsh, D. (1995). Schizotypal symptoms and signs in the Roscommon Family Study: Their factor structure and familial relationship with psychotic and affective disorders. *Archives of General Psychiatry, 52*(4), 296–303.

Lees Roitman, S. E., Cornblatt, B. A., Bergman, A., Obuchowski, M., Mitropoulou, V., Keefe, R. S. E., Silverman, J. M., & Siever, L. J. (1997). Attentional functioning in schizotypal personality disorder. *American Journal of Psychiatry, 154*, 655–660. Retrieved from https://www.researchgate.net/profile/Jeremy_Silverman/publication/14081478_Attentional_functioning_in_schizotypal_personality_disorder/links

Livesley, J. W. (2001). *Handbook of personality disorders: Theory, research, and treatment.* New York, NY: The Guilford Press.

Mayo Clinic. (2017a). Schizotypal personality disorder—Symptoms and causes. *Mayo Clinic.* Retrieved from https://www.mayoclinic .org/diseases-conditions/schizotypal-personality-disorder/symptoms -causes/syc-20353919

Mayo Clinic. (2017b). Schizotypal personality disorder—Diagnosis and treatment. *Mayo Clinic.* Retrieved from https://www.mayoclinic .org/diseases-conditions/schizotypal-personality-disorder/diagnosis -treatment/drc-20353924

Mayo Clinic Staff. (2012). Schizotypal personality disorder. *Mayo Clinic.* Archived from the original (http://www.mayoclinic.com /health/schizotypal-personality-disorder/DS00830/DSECTION=causes) on March 9, 2012. Retrieved February 21, 2012.

McGlashan T. H., Grilo, C. M., Skodol, A. E., Gunderson, J. G., Shea, M. T., Morey, L. C., Zanarini, M. C., & Stout, R. L. (2000). The collaborative longitudinal personality disorders study: Baseline axis I/ II and II/II diagnostic co-occurrence. *Acta Psychiatrica Scandinavica, 102,* 256–264.

McGuffin, P., & Thapar, A. (1992). The genetics of personality disorder. *British Journal of Psychiatry, 160,* 12–23.

Millon, T. (2004). *Personality disorders in modern life* (2nd ed.). New York, NY: Wiley.

Minichiello, W. E. (1987). Schizotypal personality disorder: A poor prognostic indicator for behavior therapy in the treatment of obsessive-compulsive disorder. *Journal of Anxiety Disorders, 1*(3), 273–276.

Mulder, R. T., Joyce, P. R., Frampton, C. M., Luty, S. E., & Sullivan, P. F. (2006). Six months of treatment for depression: outcome and predictors of the course of illness. *The American Journal of Psychiatry, 163,* 95–100.

Nigg, J. T., & Goldsmith, H. H. (1994). Genetics of personality disorders: Perspectives from personality and psychopathology research. *Psychology Bulletin, 115,* 346–380.

Psychology Today (2017). Schizotypal personality disorder. Retrieved April 8, 2018, from https://www.psychologytoday.com/conditions /schizotypal-personality-disorder

Rado, S. (1954). Dynamics and classification of disordered behavior. *American Journal of Psychiatry, 110,* 406–416.

Raine, A. (1991). The SPQ: A scale for the assessment of schizotypal personality disorder based on DSM-III-R criteria. *Schizophrenic Bulletin, 17,* 555–564.

Raine, A. (2006). Schizotypal personality: Neurodevelopmental and psychosocial trajectories. *Annual Review of Psychology, 2*, 291–326.

Schizotypal personality disorder. (2013). *Diagnostic and statistical manual of mental disorders*, Fifth Edition (DSM-5) (pp. 655–659) Washington, D.C.: American Psychiatric Association.

Siever, L. J. (1992). Schizophrenia spectrum disorders. *Review of Psychiatry, 11*, 25–42.

Skodol, A. E., Gunderson, J. G., McGlashan, T. H., Dyck, I. R., Stout, R. L., Bender, D. S., . . . Oldjam, J. M. (2002). Functional impairment in patients with schizotypal, borderline, avoidant, or obsessive-compulsive personality disorder. *American Journal of Psychiatry, 159*(2), 276–283.

Squires-Wheeler, E., Skodol, A. E., Bassett, A., & Erlenmeyer-Kimling, L. (1989). DSM-III-R schizotypal personality traits in offspring of schizophrenic disorder, affective disorder, and normal control parents. *Journal of Psychiatric Research, 23*(3–4), 229–239.

Torgersen, S., Onstad, S., Skre, I., Edvardsen, J., & Kringlen, E. (1993). "True" schizotypal personality disorder: A study of co-twins and relatives of schizophrenic probands. *American Journal of Psychiatry, 150*(11), 1661–1667.

University of Colorado Colorado Springs. (2001). An Empirical Investigation of Jung's Personality Types and Psychological Disorder Features. *Journal of Psychological Type/University of Colorado Colorado Springs*. Vol. 58, 33–36. Retrieved August 10, 2013, from

Varma, S. L., & Sharma, I. (1993). Psychiatric morbidity in the first degree relatives of schizophrenic patients. *British Journal of Psychiatry, 162*, 672–678.

WebMed. (2017). Schizotypal personality disorder facts. Retrieved May 26, 2018, from https://www.medicinenet.com/schizotypal_personality _disorder/article.htm#what_are_causes_and_risk_factors_for_schizotypal _personality_disorder

Wood, J. C. (2010). *The cognitive behavioral therapy workbook for personality disorders: A step-by-step program*. Oakland, CA: New Harbinger Publications.

Glossary

anxiety

A feeling of fear, uneasiness, and worry, often generalized, not focused. An overreaction to a situation. Anxiety disorder: An individual experiences anxiety regularly.

attachment

Any form of behavior that results in a person attaining or retaining proximity to some preferred individual, who is usually conceived as stronger and/or wiser.

bias in psychiatric diagnosis

Gender differences in psychiatric diagnosis. Possible reasons: (a) Some methodological artifacts can potentially produce differential base rates of a particular disorder in men and women, even when in reality men and women show comparable base rates of the disorder. (b) Bias on the part of clinicians might produce differential rates of false positive (or false negative) diagnoses for a particular disorder in men and women, resulting in an overestimate of sex differences in the occurrence of that disorder. (c) The nature of the diagnostic criteria themselves—the symptom criteria for a particular disorder may be constructed in such a way that the disorder will inevitably be over- or underdiagnosed in men or women (Bornstein, R. F. 1993, *The dependent personality*. New York, NY: The Guilford Press).

causal

A direct relationship between events, behavior, or stimuli where introducing one results in the other occurring.

causality

The relationship between one act and its consequence; the necessary results of the actions of one entity on another.

cluster

In psychology, one of three general categories of personality disorders—Cluster A (odd, bizarre, eccentric); Cluster B (dramatic, erratic); Cluster C (anxious, fearful).

comorbid/comorbidity

The simultaneous presence of two or more conditions or diseases in the same person.

construct

Generally, a hypothetical entity (such as intelligence) treated as though actually in existence.

defense mechanism

Response, typically unconscious, by which the ego is protected from anxiety, guilt, shame, or loss of pride.

denial

Defensive refusal to recognize external reality, emotional reactions, or motive.

depersonalization

A feeling of being disengaged from one's surroundings.

differential diagnosis

Considering all possible diagnostic categories that might be compatible with what is known about an individual's abnormality and its development.

epidemiology
Affecting, or tending to affect, many individuals within a population.

epigenesis
The notion that for an individual, there are preplanned stages of development.

fundamental distribution error
Social perceivers tend to overemphasize dispositional interpretations of others' behavior, even in the face of evidence indicating that situational pressures played a role in determining the behavior in question.

hypervigilance
An increased awareness of a person's surroundings and being constantly tense or on guard.

incidence
Rate of occurrence of new cases of a given condition in a given time period.

individuation
The process of becoming differentiated as an individual.

monozygotic twins
Twins developed from a single ovum—identical twins.

nosology
Systematic classification of disease.

paraphrenia
General term meaning abnormal, insane, psychotic thinking.

person perception
The way individuals think about, approve, and assess other individuals.

personality disorder

An enduring pattern of inner experience and behavior that deviates from the norm of the individual's culture. The pattern is seen in two or more of the following areas: cognition, affect, interpersonal functioning, or impulse control. The enduring pattern is inflexible and pervasive across a broad range of personal and social situations, beginning in the teenage years or early adulthood.

phenomenology

The study of the development of human consciousness and self-awareness as a preface of philosophy. The description of the formal structure of the objects of awareness and of awareness itself in abstraction from any claims concerning existence.

phobia

Strong fear of an unreasonable or irrational type.

physiognomy

The study of the personality as a function of the appearance of the body, especially the face.

preconscious

Area of the mind where memories exist, which can be brought readily to awareness; in between the unconscious and the conscious.

prevalence

The total frequency of a given condition at a particular moment in time.

prognosis

Prediction of the course and outcome of a disorder.

projection

Attributing certain aspects of self to others without awareness.

psychopathology

Abnormal, maladaptive behavior or mental activity.

rationalization

A plausible explanation for some behavior that comes after the decision or the act, but not the real reason.

recidivism

Repeated or habitual relapse.

reinforcement

Strengthening various behavioral responses through rewards.

splitting

Dichotomizing, such as the distinction between the good self and the bad self.

symbol

Distinguished from a sign; a "living" symbol expresses something relatively unknown to consciousness that is pregnant with meaning that cannot be characterized in any other way; formulates an essential, unconscious factor, not something already conventionally known.

symptom

A manifestation of an illness or emotional disturbance.

trait

Any more-or-less permanent aspect or characteristic of an individual; a person's reliably consistent ways of operating.

unconscious

That portion of the psyche of which one is unaware and that contains desires and drives.

Resources

Articles about personality disorders in Web4health Web site: http://web4 health.info/en/answers/border-menu.htm

Baer, R. A., Peters, J. R., Eisenlohr-Moul, T. A., Geiger, P. J., & Sauer, S. E. (2012). Emotion-related cognitive processes in borderline personality disorder: A review of the empirical literature. *Clinical Psychology Review, 32*(5), 359–369.

Bender, D. S., Dolan, R. T., Skodol, A. E., Sanislow, C. A., Dyck, I. R., McGlashan, T. H., . . . Gunderson, G. (2001). Treatment utilization by patients with personality disorders. *The American Journal of Psychiatry, 158*(2), 295–302. Published online. doi:10.1176/appi. ajp.158.2.295

Benjamin, L. S. (1996). *Interpersonal diagnosis and treatment of personality disorders* (2nd ed.). New York, NY: Guilford Press.

Costa, P. T. Jr., & Widiger, T. A. (Eds.). (1994). *Personality disorders and the five-factor model of personality*. Washington, D.C.: American Psychological Association.

Grant, B. F., Hasin, D. S., Stinson, F. S., Dawson, D. A., Chou, S. P., Ruan, W. J., & Pickering, R. P. (2004). Prevalence, correlates, and disability of personality disorders in the United States: Result from the National Epidemiologic Survey on Alcohol and Related Conditions. *The Journal of Clinical Psychiatry, 65*(7), 948–958.

Johnson, J. G., Cohen, P., & Brown, J. (1999). Childhood maltreatment increases risk for personality disorders during early adulthood. *Archives of General Psychiatry, 56*(7), 600–606.

Kernberg, O. F. (1975). *Borderline conditions and pathological narcissism*. New York, NY: Jason Aronson.

Leichsenring, F., & Leibing, E. (2003). The effectiveness of psychodynamic and cognitive behavior therapy in the treatment of personality disorders: A meta-analysis. *American Journal of Psychiatry, 190,* 80. *Focus.* Published online July 1, 2005. doi:10.1176/foc.3.3.417

Leutgeb, V., Wabnegger, A., Leitner, M., Zussner T., Scharmüller, W., Klug, D., & Schienle, A. (2016). Altered cerebellar-amygdala connectivity in violent offenders: A resting-state fMRI study. *Neuroscience Letters, 1*(610), 160–164.

Lieb, K., Zanarini, M. C., Schmahl, C., Linehan, M. M., & Bohus, M. (2004). Borderline personality disorder. *The Lancet, 364*(9432), 453–461.

Livesley, John W. (2003). *Practical management of personality disorder.* New York, NY: The Guilford Press.

Loranger, A. W., Sartorius, N., Andreoli, A., Berger, P., Buchheim, P., Channabasavanna, S. M. . . . & Ferguson, B. (1994). The International Personality Disorder Examination: The World Health Organization/ Alcohol, Drug Abuse, and Mental Health Administration International Pilot Study of Personality Disorders. *Archives of General Psychiatry, 51*(3), 215–224.

Millon, T. (2004). *Personality disorders in modern life* (2nd ed.). New York, NY: Wiley.

Phillips, K. A., & McElroy, S. L. (2000). Personality disorders and traits in patients with body dysmorphic disorder. *Comprehensive Psychiatry, 41*(4), 229–236.

Plakun, E. M., Burkhardt, P. E., & Müller, J. P. (1985). 14-year follow-up of borderline and schizotypal personality disorders. *Comprehensive Psychiatry, 26*(7) 448–455.

Pozza, A., Domenichetti, S., Mazzoni, G. P., & Dettore, D. (2016). The comorbidity of cluster C personality disorders in obsessive compulsive disorder as a marker of anxiety and depression severity. *European Psychiatry, 33*(Supplement), S202–S203.

Skodol, A. C. (2011). Personality disorder types proposed for DSM-5. *Journal of Personality Disorders, 25*(2), 150.

Tielbeek, J., Medland, S. E., Benyamin, B., Byrne, E. M., Heath, A. C., Madden, P. A., … Verweij, K. J. (2012). Unraveling the genetic etiology of adult antisocial behavior: A genome-wide association study. *PloS ONE, 7(10),* e45086.

Winnicott, D. (2012). *Playing and reality* (pp. 26–38). London: Routledge Classics.

Resource Web Sites and Organizations

American Psychological Association (APA), www.apa.org
Based in Washington, D.C., the American Psychological Association is a scientific and professional organization that represents psychology in the

United States. It is the largest association of psychologists worldwide. Its mission is to advance the creation, communication, and application of psychological knowledge to benefit society and improve people's lives.

BetterHelp, https://www.betterhelp.com/advice/personality-disorder /what-is
This organization provides a description of each disorder with symptoms, diagnosis, treatment plan, statistics, and online connection with a licensed therapist.

International Society for Mental Health Online (ISMHO), www.ismho .org
An international community exploring and promoting mental health in the digital age. Its members include students, teachers, researchers, clinical practitioners, and others interested in using Internet technologies to sustain positive mental health.

Mayo Clinic, https://www.mayoclinic.org/diseases-conditions/personality -disorders/symptoms-causes/syc
This site provides information on diseases and conditions, Mayo Clinic campuses, symptoms, patient and visitor guide, doctor and medical staff, "contact us."

Mental Health America (MHA), www.nmha.org/gov/information/get -info/personality-disorders
MHA is one of the country's leading nonprofits dedicated to helping people live emotionally healthier lives.

National Alliance on Mental Illness, www.nami.org
As the nation's largest grassroots mental health organization, it is dedicated to improving the lives of persons living with serious mental illness, along with their families, through advocacy, research, support, and education.

National Association for Cognitive-Behavioral Therapists (NACBT), www.nacbt.org
The leading organization dedicated exclusively to supporting, teaching, and developing cognitive-behavioral therapy and those who practice it. Laypeople can direct many questions about CBT to the site and request information on how to find a CBT therapist in their area.

National Institute of Mental Health (NIMH), www.nimh.gov
The mission of NIMH is to transform the understanding and treatment of mental illnesses through basic and clinical research, paving the way for prevention, recovery, and cure.

Psych Central, https://psychcentral.com/disorders/, and J. Grohol, http://psychcentral.com
Information about different conditions and disorders, drugs, current news, and research and books about mental health, online screening tests for certain disorders, and relationship questions. There is an "Ask the Therapist" section, a community discussion board, and "The Exhausted Woman" blog.

http://psychcentral.com/resources
A comprehensive guide to mental and emotional resources for sufferers and their families, featuring hundreds of links and informative articles.

Psychology Today, https://www.psychologytoday.com/conditions/
Find profiles of therapists, support groups, and books. This site offers the latest from the world of psychology, behavioral research, practical guidance, and basics information.

ScienceDirect, http://www.sciencedirect.com
Information about journals, articles, and book chapters.

Index

About the Author

VERA SONJA MAASS, PHD, is a licensed clinical psychologist, a marriage and family therapist, and a mental health counselor in private practice in Indianapolis, Indiana. She holds professional memberships in the American Psychological Association, the Indiana Psychological Association, and the American Counseling Association. Her teaching experience includes terms as adjunct faculty at the University of Indianapolis and Ivy Tech Community College. Maass is the author of eight books: *Understanding Social Anxiety: A Recovery Guide for Sufferers, Family, and Friends* (Praeger, 2017); *Finding Love That Lasts: Breaking the Pattern of Dead End Relationships* (Rowman & Littlefield, 2012); *Coping with Control and Manipulation: Making the Difference Between Being a Target and Becoming a Victim* (Praeger, 2010); *The Cinderella Test: Would You Really Want the Shoe to Fit? Subtle Ways Women Are Seduced and Socialized into Servitude and Stereotypes* (Praeger, 2009); *Lifestyle Changes* (Routledge, 2008); *Facing the Complexities of Women's Sexual Desire* (Springer Science + Business Media, 2007); *Women's Group Therapy* (Springer, 2002/2006); and *Counseling Single Parents* (Springer, 2000).